UNLEASH YOUR CRAZY TO WIN

Disclaimer: Some names and identifying details have been changed to protect the privacy of individuals.

Printed and bound in Canada at McNally Robinson Booksellers.
1120 Grant Avenue, Winnipeg, Manitoba R3M 2A6.

Second Edition, 2016

Cover design by Garry Blatz.
Book design by McNally Robinson Booksellers.

Cover photograph by Adeline Loewen.

www.mcnallyrobinson.com/selfpublishing

ISBN 978-1-77280-028-9

UNLEASH YOUR CRAZY TO WIN

How Overcoming Infertility Led to Business Success

VICKI OLATUNDUN

To Victor,

What did I do in my life to deserve you?

You are the man that made calling me mom possible

I love you.

Contents

Foreword

I wanted to reword 'foreword' to 'forward' … that's much more of a 'Vicki' word, and you will find this book full of 'Vicki' kind of words. You will love that she does not use a passive word when a bold one will do. I am privileged to provide you some thoughts not only on the book, the story, the principles, but ultimately upon the author and the remarkable relevance of what she shares.

I have come to know Vicki as many things. She is passionate – powerful – a crusader for the underdog – courageous and fiercely determined. She truly is 'a dragon slayer' and a force to be reckoned with. I have known her for well over a decade and can assure you that there is nothing half-way, lukewarm, or mediocre about her. I have been with her on team projects when she leans in to make a point and stress a matter of significance – and it isn't surprising to find that she trained to be a lawyer. I have seen her take on the needs of the homeless and the helpless and, with all the tenacity of a bulldog, she presses and perseveres until help is provided and hope is given. I have been in meetings, public and private, where the stakes are high and the tension tangible and she steps up to speak in the clear, articulate and measured fashion of her British upbringing – and you can't help but pause, listen and breathe again.

But when she begins to talk about her children all the powerful images fade away and she re-emerges with all the whimsical wonder that characterizes those who have experienced the miracle of bringing life into this world. It has always struck me how contrasting were the natures of this woman – and it wasn't until I read this book that it all made sense.

It is appropriate that the first part of her book is the personal story of infertility – the practical people will want to skip to the application – resist the urge – the application has so much more meaning with this as the backdrop. As I read the introduction I found people coming to mind who need to hear the honesty of the pain that is associated with the news of barrenness. My thoughts automatically turned to a young family acquaintance who in a moment of vulnerability shared with my wife and I that she had just found out this same diagnosis. There was a tangible ache in her voice as she attempted to make the message sound somehow less stark and final. *We will never be able to have children.* Immersed in those words of fact was a truck load of grief over the death of hopes, dreams, marvels and miracles. I was suddenly very aware how important and yet how incredibly difficult it was for this young woman to say those words. My heart aches for her and her husband – they would make such great parents. In all of that, I didn't know what to say, how to comfort or console. There is something about the effect of this diagnosis that runs deeper than ego and our sense of self. It causes the spirit of men and women to, like clams, slam shut and hide away this most numbing news. For all of them this book comes to at least say: *"You are not alone – someone understands this deep hole in your life."* It also might just spur them on to paint a room yellow with optimism! I found myself laughing out loud as she named her first chapter 'round one' … that is so like Vicki.

The second half of the book moves on and applies the lessons to practical application. Even here the lessons are those which have been etched and hammered out in the toughest place of all – the flesh and blood experiences of life. Her courage shows through in that she does not skirt the difficult passages. The release from the shelter was not just an inconvenient set back – it was a blow that could very easily have finished her. Her work there was, for her, deeply personal and not just a job. She was there during critical times in the life of the organization and by sheer determination she was a part of keeping the ship afloat. The extent of her integrity is that she includes this in the story when it would be so easy to pass it over. But failure in one area of life is not final – and that is the grist that is a part of the call to perspective. If there was any doubt to her humanity this was a time that revealed that, as with all of us, our limits and boundaries. Tears and fears and skyrocketing blood pressure, and mourning for what was lost were all a part of this season. Don't assume that the lessons of the book are theoretical.

The ten points outlined in this second part of the book can serve as a template and model for accomplishing great and crazy things! An elderly saint used to say to me: *There is no happenstance in the will of God.* I have often thought of that statement in light of Vicki's remarkable leadership with Anna's House. We have often talked about how the lessons and work at the shelter were ideal preparation for her to assume leadership at Anna's House. And her heart for children and families seems such a natural blending of passions. And God's will always calls for obedience and a craziness that is willing to step out and risk for a hope that is greater than just our own need. May those of you who read this story … and apply these lessons … discover that in your own endeavors as well.

Respectfully,
Dr. Larry Dahl
District Superintendent, Church of the Nazarene

Preface

Victory is always possible for the person who refuses to stop fighting.

– Napoleon Hill

I have searched bookstore shelves for quite a while and not found any books that really explain or express the many feelings that come with the diagnosis of infertility, at least none that spoke to me.

Infertility is a tough experience and I now understand why many people who go through it are often too devastated and disappointed to talk about their infertility. Not only is it painful — it screams failure at you. I found it very difficult to talk to others about my experience when I was going through it. A diagnosis can start you on a very lonely road filled with insensitive comments, uncompassionate people and shame. I can almost understand the insensitive people and silly comments; when people don't understand an issue they can say stupid things. But the feeling of shame makes no sense.

It is devastating enough to have to deal with the prospect of broken dreams and trashed hopes without also feeling bulldozed by the devastation and deep hurt that shame brings. I have no idea why exactly shame comes into the picture. I have often wondered why society seems to have created a "box of shame" for anything that is not "normal." It is normal for human beings to have sex, get pregnant and have babies. But if you cannot, it feels as though you wear a badge of shame and should be confined to the farthest corner of Outer Siberia and carry the deep pain with you for the rest of your life as punishment. Really? Why?

This doesn't make sense. Infertility is a medical condition, plain and simple. Who would inflict shame on a person diagnosed with breast cancer, ALS or MS? Then why infertility? All the diagnosis means is that your reproductive organs are not working properly. It could be for a plethora of reasons, from being born that way to the side effects of medication. But getting the diagnosis, and then having experts hand you bad news everywhere you turn, can be lonely, humiliating and discouraging.

Well, along the way I took a stand and I chose to challenge the experts and the status quo and I got the results I wanted. My hope in writing this book is to shine the light on what it feels like to be handed the box of shame while standing in the middle of that lonely road and how I fought back. It is also to share with those who have no clue the pain and the pressure that come with the experience of infertility, while also being a voice for those who find themselves standing in the middle of that lonely road.

No one chooses infertility, I didn't. It was thrown at me and rather than duck I caught it. I never thought it would become a platform for me but I decided not to hide under it but stand on the platform and use it to help. The global statistics make it clear that one in six couples deal with infertility, if my math is correct that is over half a billion people, yet we still can't talk about it. We still don't know how to talk to people who are going through it. We don't know what to say or how to say it. The stigma is real. Any other disease with this kind of number would have been considered a pandemic or an epidemic, this on the other hand is a global catastrophe and the conversation about this matter is not happening as often it could be. This book is the beginning of a conversation that needs to be had. Hello…I'm…

I found much encouragement from the stories of other families, and I say families, not just women. Men go through infertility too. They struggle too. They are either going through it by themselves or as a partner to a woman going through it or both at the same time. I hope you find comfort, courage and hope in the pages ahead as you follow me through the highs, the lows, the tears, the laughter and the eventual joy I came to experience on my journey.

For those of you going through this now, for those of you that have been through this in the past and for those of you that may find yourself about to go through this.

I get it.

I hurt with you.

I see you.

I hear you.

I stand with you.

I dare you to see there is still hope and I dare you to believe it. Your journey may not be the same as mine but I hope you will find courage in the story of my path despite the twists and turns and dead ends.

I pushed through the infertility door; this book is my way of leaving a wedge wide enough for you to push open your door. All I ask is that when you come through, do the same for others who will need to hear your story too.

Part two of the book is a little unusual, it puts you in the passenger seat of a business adventure I took using principles I learned in part one. I discovered that principles are principles and they operate in every area of life. Success is available in any kind of business and is possible if the principles are applied correctly.

Part ONE

Introduction

"I hate to be the bearer of bad news Vicki," my gynecologist said quietly. "The test results are back and they show you will never be able to have a child."

NEVER.

That was my rude and sudden introduction to infertility, a stranger that I didn't care to meet. Well, whether I liked it or not the handshake had been made and this stranger had not only banged on my door but without an invitation had moved into my house!

What do you do when someone uninvited barges past you at the door and takes up residence in your life without your permission? It was a cold, harsh and completely shocking entrance into a world I didn't even know existed — the world of infertility. It felt like jumping onto a very scary roller coaster ride in pitch-black darkness. Those very simple words from a trusted doctor literally blew my world apart. My dreams of raising a family were gone in less than twenty seconds!

My Hiroshima!

Boom!

Nothing can prepare you for such a thing.

The devastation and disappointment, the sense of failure was not made any easier by the further news that even in vitro fertilization (IVF) was not an option. I didn't qualify for any fertility treatment because my medical history included matters that made my situation very complicated; needless to say, I was medically precluded. The conclusion was NEVER and I was the medical evidence to back it.

Did I miss the last page of Cinderella, Rapunzel and Sleeping Beauty? The last lines were always "and they lived happily ever after." What happened to my fairy tale?

Those words from my doctor shattered my happy life into a million pieces.

All my hopes and dreams of having a family were dashed. In those few seconds, my "happily ever after" was snatched away from me. There was no knight in shining armour coming to rescue me, because he was already standing next to me. This tsunami hit us both — my husband and me — head on, in the face.

I could hear the words over and over. NEVER...NEVER... NEVER...

"I was innocent!" Only I could hear the screams in my head. I had done nothing wrong, but here I was pronounced legally childless with a life sentence of infertility handed down with no opportunity to appeal or be paroled... EVER.

I was thirty-seven years old. I had been happily married for ten years. I was hurt, traumatized. Why me? What did I do to anyone? As I sat there, the pain was incredible; life had hit hard and I was down for the count.

In that same moment, as I heard the countdown 10...9...8... I knew I had a choice. 7...6...5... I could lie down and play dead and accept the impending verdict 4...3...2... or FIGHT....

Welcome to Round One.

Round ONE

If you fight you might lose- if you don't you already have.

– Bertholt Brecht

It all started early fall 2001 when my friend Marcia called. She wanted us to hang out and grab a coffee. This was nothing out of the ordinary for us. So, as usual we chatted excitedly for a few minutes about this and that. Then, she said she had a hunch... one of those girly intuition things; she wanted me to go and see a gynecologist. My hot, flavoured coffee suddenly turned cold and sour. I thought what? Why? Who wants to do that if it's not absolutely necessary? But she wouldn't let it go. As most good girlfriends do, she kept going on and on and on.

I left the café thinking what in the world had she been smoking? But she pushed, she called, texted, phoned and left the clinic's number. She was stalking me; she was in my face. By the end of the week I had had enough, so just to shut her up I called the clinic mid-November and booked an appointment for some time in January 2002, the earliest I could get. To this day I am not sure how I got the appointment because I found out later that you had to be referred by a doctor and I didn't have one at the time. I got the appointment anyhow.

Mid-January I went in for the appointment and the doctor politely asked why I was there. I felt a little silly so I chuckled and said, "To check that all the plumbing is working." So he proceeded to examine my abdomen and within twenty seconds he said, "We can take out the tumour, no problem." I thought what are you talking about? I came here for a general checkup, what tumour? He explained that I had a huge fibroid tumour in my uterus and that they could not take it out immediately because it was too big. They would have to put my body into temporary menopause for three months to shrink it to an operable size. Huh?

I was shocked, stunned; I could barely move. My immediate reaction was denial. I walked into that office a happy-go-lucky human and within seconds I was dealing with having to have major surgery. No. I didn't believe him. I didn't hear another word. I couldn't. It was like a movie... everything unfolding in slow motion and then the words hit me like bullets.

All kinds of questions flashed through my mind. Is the tumour malignant? Am I going to die? Menopause? Would this lead to a hysterectomy?

I was troubled. It was surreal. It is weird how life can change so quickly without warning. I rushed out of the clinic with tear-filled eyes and burst out crying when I got into the car. My thoughts were running 100 kmh. I turned on the radio. I turned it to the highest volume; I was trying to drown out all the wild thoughts that were running through my mind. I had tears streaming down my face and my heart was sad. I was driving back to the office in tears, praying that I would not kill anyone because I could barely see the road. I had never had surgery before and this was something I had not anticipated, I was in total shock. I had no idea what this all meant. How I got back to the office that day I will never know. I had to dry my tears and put on a brave face when I got back to work and it was business as usual until home time. I held it in and blurted it all out to Victor when he got home. He was very supportive and he agreed we needed a second opinion.

Marcia's hunch was right and when I called her even she was in shock. She had what I call a "niggly." Sometimes there is something that bothers you, it niggles you. Don't ignore it. Call it intuition, gut feeling, whatever; don't push it aside. It could make a big difference for you or someone else.

I was still reeling. In reaction I did one of the most important things I could ever have done — I called my "NASCAR" team. I had just suffered a major blowout and I needed a team around me who could help ease the shock and get me back on the road, back in the race quickly. When life hits it is so easy to run and hide or fall off a cliff or become depressed. I believe everyone should have a NASCAR team. For me it was six very close friends I turned to, including my husband, sister and mentor.

I talked with them all individually, and sometimes with two or three together; I developed a game plan based on their advice and got my mind back on track. It was literally like a whole crew all over a car during a pit stop in the Daytona 500.

When life hits you in the face you have a choice, you can

become depressed and discouraged, which for most people is a natural bent, or you can fight it. I was very tempted to just lie on the floor in the fetal position and cry, but I asked myself "what good would that do?"

I did what I knew to do. I used my faith, family and friends to help me. Strategy will always triumph over strength. When stuff like this hits the fan you need support. Life was never designed be a solo sport.

The first thing that happened was that my fears were allayed. I had a flat tire... rather than a slashed one. I calmed down and did some research and found out what a fibroid tumour actually was. What I had was not malignant. I made the decision to go for a second opinion and they confirmed the original diagnosis.

In real estate or a new business they say *Location, Location, Location* is the biggest factor; with medical issues it is *Information, Information, Information.* I talked to women who had had the operation I was planning to have. I found as much information as I possibly could. I read magazines, books, periodicals, white papers, journals — you name it, I read it. I found testimonials, stories of women who were going through the same thing, and it really helped to keep me in a positive state of mind.

I found out that putting my body into menopause was temporary and things would eventually go back to normal. Was there the possibility of a hysterectomy? Yes, but I was going to focus on what I could control. Was I worried? Yes. Was I powerless? No! They say that worry is the interest you pay for trouble that has not yet happened to you. I had paid enough.

The operation was scheduled for June 27, 2002. I did all I could to live life normally until then. In the meantime, Victor and I were in the process of buying a new home, our first home. It was a cute little house in a quiet part of town. It needed a little renovating as it was quite dated, and I have to say that it was a well-needed distraction. It was very exciting that we were finally buying a home.

It was mid-March and we had an evening appointment with our lawyers to exchange all the final paper work. Victor and I had discussed a few things at lunch earlier in the day. We were completely thrilled. We had waited for this day a long time and it was finally here. We kissed each other goodbye at 1:00 p.m. and both went back to work.

At 2:30 p.m. Victor showed up at my office again. I thought he had forgotten something. He quietly explained that his company was restructuring; the same company that had brought us here from the UK two years earlier had just downsized him. We had a decision to make. We could react or respond. We both knew what was going on. It was just life. We burst out laughing and prayed, and decided to keep our evening appointment and buy our home. We had wisely based our home-buying capacity on my sole income, as I was the lower earner but it would still be a stretch. It was a little scary, the prospect of a new home with only one income. We have both always believed that faith is spelled R. I. S. K., so we took a leap of faith. We exchanged paperwork and bought our home that day.

The day of the operation was coming up soon; nothing had changed physically. I took my medication and just lived. I was obviously a little anxious. I had those odd thoughts like everyone else contemplating major surgery — completely off thoughts that I was going to die... random thoughts from nowhere. But I refused to let my mind go there. I had informed my office about the operation and recovery time, which was twelve weeks. So all was good, or so I thought.

I decided to work up until the day of the surgery. I had spoken to the person in charge of our human resources and explained all my plans and all was agreed but on June 25, which was two days before the operation, my boss called me into his office for a quick meeting. We had a few new projects we were working on and I figured he was going to be asking me about where I had left things. We talked about various things, he then asked about Victor's employment. I explained that he had just been downsized. All of a sudden the conversation changed and the atmosphere grew cold and immediately after that he told me I was terminated. What? I was shocked to say the least, I felt hurt and betrayed. It was very bad timing. New home, husband unemployed; now I was unemployed and facing major surgery in two days. It is very easy to move from hurt to angry and offended but I chose to respond in a completely different way.

Instead, the next day I bought flowers and chocolates for my colleagues and now former bosses; I forgave any wrongs, cleaned out my desk and left. Tough stuff but it had to be done. Trust me, I felt like doing quite the opposite but how could I go into major surgery with all that on my mind?

The next day came quickly and I was anxious... I am quite a house-proud person and I like to have a neat and organized home. Usually I would tidy everything in the morning before my day starts. In response to how I was feeling about dying, I deliberately left a mess. I told my husband that I would be back to clean it up.

The myomectomy went as well as could be expected. They removed an 8 lb. fibroid tumour from my uterus. I had a Caesarean-like scar on my abdomen; my OB/GYN said it was a "smile" shape. It didn't matter; it was still painful. It was really odd having a Caesarean-type operation with no baby to show for it. The pain after the operation was nothing like I had ever felt before. It was tough; I felt the most pain when I coughed and when I sneezed I thought my brain would fall out! Apparently I had lots of little fibroid tumours; they took out the biggest one and left in all the tiny ones to avoid further complications. I was so relieved that they were not forced to do a hysterectomy because I wanted children. I went home to tidy up like I had promised and spent the next few months recuperating.

The follow-up appointment a few weeks later came quickly and I found out that my uterus was intact but the lining was left paper-thin. I didn't think too much about that at the time, but it would play a very significant role later on.

Victor and I had wanted to start a family but we just weren't getting pregnant. I thought that it had been the fibroid tumours that had prevented us from getting pregnant all along. So I spent the rest of 2002 recovering, looking forward to things going back to normal and the possibility of starting a family. The next year we went back to the clinic for more checkups. We were still not pregnant and we wanted to know why. A slew of tests began, on me and on Victor. I had to take my temperature at the same time every day and log it, and monitor my monthly cycle. Test results came back; I was not ovulating. If I was not ovulating then there was no way I could get pregnant. That was the first piece of bad news; then came a further blow. My FSH (follicle stimulating hormone) levels were at 13. To get pregnant one's FSH levels need to be at 10 or below.

It was at this point that my doctor delivered the ultimate blow. He explained that during the myomectomy he had removed so much of my uterine lining in order to get the fibroid tumour that there was barely anything left. He said that if by some impossible way I ever became pregnant I would never be able to carry to term and certainly not give birth naturally. Then my doctor told me our dreams of having a family were over, we were infertile and most importantly there was nothing that modern medicine could do to fix it. Up until then I did not have any reason to consider the question of infertility. Why would I? I had heard of only one other person who had fertility challenges and that was because she had polycystic fibrosis. Everyone else in my world got pregnant when they wanted to. As with things of this nature, the questions came a thousand per second. What does this mean? What do I tell my family? Am I really barren? What are the options now? How do I tell my in-laws? Those inaudible questions in my head were screaming so loudly in that quiet little office I was worried the receptionist could hear them at the front desk.

My doctor sensitively explained other options we had. It boiled down to surrogacy or adoption and/or embryo adoption and even these for us were tenuous. These were all well and good and for many who have had children by these means I celebrate them. (One of our friends out of the blue actually offered to be a surrogate for us.) A family can be created in so many ways but deep down I wanted to physically give birth to my own children and considering my situation it was easy to think it was not possible anymore.

Many years prior, while sitting in a church meeting, I heard a quote that touched my mind and reminded me that crazy was an essential ingredient to making the impossible possible.

> *The reasonable man adapts himself to the world; the unreasonable one persists in trying to adapt the world to himself. Therefore, all progress depends on the unreasonable man.*
>
> —George Bernard Shaw
>
> *Irish dramatist & socialist (1856 - 1950)*

For some reason, I have never forgotten it and it plays a key role in the way I "do life" today. The word "unreasonable" can be defined as "not governed by reason, irrational or absurd," or "exceeding reasonable limits."

In very plain language, my interpretation of what Shaw said is that all progress depends on the crazy person. After that I decided to stop being "reasonable." It was no different now.

From the light bulb to the test tube baby, every great inventor had people who said their idea or vision was crazy. I think of Orville & Wilbur Wright who dreamed of flying and invented a machine in 1903. Their dream would have seemed ridiculous at the time but the brothers were determined and focused and they made it happen. Today, we all fly in aeroplanes without a thought because to us it's now our normal.

How about Martin Cooper? He dreamed of a phone that could be as mobile as people. At that time it was a crazy idea. He designed the first cell phone way back in 1973 after years of trials. The first mobile phone cost $3900 USD and cost 50 cents a minute to talk. The average person could not afford one; now virtually everyone has a cell phone and many phones have apps that allow communication across the world for free! Who would have thought that possible? His crazy has become our normal.

The position I took regarding my infertility, despite the diagnosis, was regarded as pretty crazy. I couldn't accept the diagnosis. I just couldn't. That would have been the reasonable thing to do but if I did, then nothing would have changed. I had made up my mind and there was no going back. I was about to make life adapt to me, despite the odds — I was almost thirty-seven years old with a medical history that was not great, having had a myomectomy.

I dreamed of having a family, I believed the impossible could happen. In order for my dream to become reality I had no other option than to join the elite club of those crazy dreamers who had gone before me and live my own dream.

Round TWO

When something is important enough, you do it even if the odds are not in your favour.

– Elon Musk

While growing up most little girls are fascinated with princesses, Disneyesque dreams of the white dress, Prince Charming and the fairy tale castle. Wonderful endings are all too familiar — the good guys win and the bad guys lose, the dragon is slain and the damsel in distress is rescued. But all too often reality is stark in contrast to all that we have imagined.

In reality, often the Wicked Witch of the West does not get banished from the kingdom but moves in next door, and today the needle that pricked Sleeping Beauty is not in a spindle — it's in the constant barrage of advertising that keeps us comparing ourselves to the next super model — now we actually *want* to sleep, in protest. Hello Prozac.

That is not to say that I didn't have fragments of the fairy tale — sometimes I got a few pages of the fairy tale — and there were many times when a few paragraphs of "happily ever after" showed up, but other times several pages of my fairy tale were ripped out and replaced with parts of a horror story.

I was never really a goodie-two-shoes kind of girl growing up but I still behaved myself most of the time. I was the house captain and school prefect, but I was not perfect.

There is still the notion of the "good girl" out there. They do all that their parents ask (not always, if only they knew…), graduate from high school, rush off to university, graduate at twenty, and then head off to law school. They meet the handsome post-graduate, fall in love and get married after a whirlwind romance and have 2.4 kids and a dog. There is the new house, two new cars and great jobs. And life is peachy...

Not quite.

Nobody mentions the periods of unemployment, the times of illness, and the in-law visits, disagreements, money management issues and Cornflakes! (Yes, Victor and I fought about breakfast cereals.) But it wasn't all doom and gloom — there were many memorable and fun times but the journey was never as we imagined; sometimes it was more fascinating, quite "novelesque," and at other times, OMG!

I was no different from any other little girl. I had dreams and I did marry the Knight in Shining Armour, a sapodilla-brown, gorgeous, chocolate man. He was a kind, generous, God-fearing gentle giant, a "brainiac" too, a scientist who loves and plays basketball. There is no doubt in my mind that I won the husband lottery! (I will never forget one of our first dates. His team was playing basketball in a local league, I was sitting in the bleachers and I overheard two girls discussing how cute number 23 was, rock solid muscle and a cute butt and an amazing player. I wanted to say "Mine!")

But here I was hand in hand with the knight and the dragon in front of us was huge and even I knew that a tiny little sword would not be enough. It was like being on a raft and facing a tsunami.

All I wanted was a baby. It didn't seem like an unreasonable request. Was that too much to ask?

The diagnosis of infertility was hard to accept, it was horrible; it was so painful because it was so final. Victor and I were told our dreams really were over but I refused to accept it. All the odds were stacked against us and our stack of odds was high — everything I knew was in the way, medical history, ethnicity, age and more. It was so unfair. There were so many people who had babies and literally threw them away. There is an African proverb, "He that has a head has no hat and he that has a hat has no head." In our situation it meant there were those of us who wanted children and couldn't have them and there were those who had them and didn't want them, the irony of life. I have been a fighter most of my life but this fight was huge and I didn't have the foggiest idea where to start.

When our doctor delivered the news to us, he sat with us for a few minutes sharing our pain. We could tell he hurt with us and for us. He was one of those people who did what they were designed to do. He was born to be a gynecologist; he had a bedside manner that was sensitive and calming. He was really sad to give us the news but he legally had no choice. As we got up to leave, he hugged me and just as we said our goodbyes he said, "I don't know why I am telling you this but I feel I have to." He then told us about a patient he had had the previous year. Her case was also hopeless, even worse than mine. Her FSH levels were at 65 — off the charts (mine were 13 going on 15). He said he remembered delivering the same kind of news to her and she promised to come back the next year pregnant. She did. He had no scientific or medical reason for how she got pregnant.

That was all the hope I needed — that sliver of hope to add faith to. That was enough to help me believe it was possible, I now had proof. It was real to me; right there and then faith and hope arose inside and I took a stand. Without hope it is impossible to dream or even imagine possibilities. I was determined to be the story he told to the next devastated couple. As we left I said "Hasta la vista doc." He smiled empathetically but from the look on his face we could tell that even though he had told us the patient's story he didn't have much hope for us.

It was a lot to take in. As we left, Victor did not know what to say to me. We got into the car after the appointment and you could have heard a pin drop in the middle of midday traffic. There was nothing to say. After what seemed like forever, he asked me where I wanted to go. Without missing a beat I said "Home Depot." He looked puzzled. He repeated the question and I repeated the answer. An awkward silence followed. He later told me that he was thinking "I married you because you were a little crazy, now you have absolutely lost your mind" ... and might I add, understandably so. Devastation does crazy things to the mind.

My thoughts were a million miles away....

If you are a boxing fan you might remember February 10, 1990 the fight between Mike Tyson and Buster Douglas. It was the first time Tyson had ever been knocked out and defeated. Up until that point he had been invincible, no one had beaten him, but after that loss everyone knew he was beatable. It was the same thing with the four-minute mile. Before Roger Bannister no one thought it was possible to run a mile in under four minutes. Well ... after he broke the record, many others broke it too — in fact the current world record is three minutes forty-three seconds. The story our doctor told me about his patient had the same effect. Infertility could be beaten; if it could happen for her it could happen for me too. But I could only hear the doctor's words of the diagnosis echo over and over and it felt like a death sentence; it was I who would have to live through it for the rest of my life. I felt I had to respond and I needed Home Depot to help me. The drive there was in complete silence. When we arrived, I jumped out of the car and I walked straight to the paint section.

It was like I had a GPS navigator attached to my shoulder. I was on a mission. I couldn't see anything else around me. I hovered over a few paint chips, then Eureka! I found it! The brightest can of yellow paint I had ever seen. All honeybees would have been proud — Winnie the Pooh yellow. It was really shockingly bright. Bear in mind my home was decorated in very inviting taupes and complementary colour-coordinated warm grey undertones. There was no place for such a colour — not even in our garage! It would have been like putting graffiti art on the side of Buckingham Palace. Victor finally broke his silence...

He asked me if I was OK. I think he was worried that I had

finally tipped over an edge. He knew I was a very out-of-the-box thinker, but this was downright crazy! I confirmed that I was OK. They say, "desperate does as desperate is" — in my case it was "crazy does as crazy is."

The difference between a mama and a bulldog is lipstick; the difference between a wannabe mama and a bulldog is none!

I explained to my nervous husband that I hated the feeling of powerlessness. It's one thing to be hit and fall down — it's quite another to not be able to ever get up. I was down and I was going to try my hardest to get up. My DNA couldn't stand it. It went against everything I knew to be true. Nothing was impossible. I had always lived that way and this situation was no different. The doctor could not have the final say. I had to respond. I had never shut my mouth my whole life and I wasn't going to start then. The only way I knew how to fight was to believe and act like the impossible was possible. The paint was the first instalment of my response.

My natural fighting modus operandi was to revisit past victories when I had to face a challenge. I wandered through the corridors of my mind and dusted off the victory files. I relived the memories of winning. I went to the victory warehouse and dug up as much as I could. There was no infertility file, as I had never faced it before.

So I did the next best thing. I put up my fists. This was definitely a David and Goliath situation. I felt outnumbered by the facts, overwhelmed by the evidence and ill-equipped by the science but like David, I had faced tough situations before and had come through. I was determined to win. I had nothing to lose, but this enemy was invisible.

How do you fight an invisible man? You pour yellow paint on him!

I arrived home from Home Depot and immediately started converting my office into a nursery. Crazy? Absolutely.

I went about it with so much joy. I bought baby magazines and cut out pictures of cute nurseries. I bought clothes for twin children because that was what I wanted. I got toys and all sorts of baby things. Out went the office desk and in came a rocking chair. I tried to paint the rocking chair in the garage but it was too cold, forty degrees below zero! I didn't realize that it was too cold for the paint and I didn't care to know, that's how crazy I was. Who in their right mind would try painting a rocking chair in such weather? I was on a mission.

I stencilled Winnie the Pooh, Piglet and Tigger all around the room. A friend gave me a crib and change table. It took about a month, but finally the nursery was ready! I told my husband that I wanted to be ready so that if someone came to the house with a baby I would be ready to receive it.

Every day I would open the nursery and the colour would shock me… and remind me of my dream to have a family. I would stand there and visualize having a baby. I know it sounds crazy, but there *was* nothing sane about my situation. Our friends would visit and when I showed them the nursery they would give me that look. I was used to it. (I am sure I barely escaped a visit from mental health.) It would get really awkward if their children fell asleep. I would offer to put them in our crib. They would politely ask if I was OK about it, they didn't want to offend me, but to me it was practice! I kept saying to myself, "that will be *my* baby soon." I got involved in every baby shower that I could. I bought really nice presents. I had fun shopping. This would be me soon.

I spent time researching stories of women who were in my situation, sentenced to a life of infertility and who eventually had children. God bless the Internet. I found so many wonderful stories that encouraged my heart. Childlessness was my current situation; it was not my definition. I didn't let the diagnosis define me. I couldn't. There were many reasons why, one of them was cultural.

It would be very difficult to tell my story without mentioning the cultural issue. It is a context that needs to be mentioned because it plays a huge role for families that have either immigrated to the West or those of a non-Western heritage. The cultural dynamics have a huge impact on infertility. I was born and raised in the UK but my heritage is African, Nigerian to be precise, and specifically from the Yoruba people.

Yorubas love children and statistics show that they are also the world's largest producer of twin children. They see lots of children as a blessing, a sign of wealth and a sign of health. So much so that wives-to-be in some parts of Yorubaland are required to be pregnant before the traditional marriage ceremony can take place. The stigma attached to infertility is awful on a completely different level.

According to Roland Hallgren in his book, *The Good Things in Life: A Study of the Traditional Religious Culture of the Yoruba People*, "Traditional Yoruba culture would plead for an abundance of three good things in life (for a man): wealth, women and children."

Despite the fact that I was born and raised and have lived in the West for most of my life, the stigma of infertility was able to find me like it had a homing device.

According to Winny Koster-Oyekan, an associate at the Women's Health and Action Research Centre, Lagos, Nigeria, a student when questioned about infertility responded negatively by saying "A woman without a child has no reason for living and will always be unhappy."

Koster-Oyekan's article, "Infertility Among Yoruba Women: Perceptions on Causes, Treatments and Consequences" makes for an interesting read on the cultural impact of infertility. Although her research was limited to women in Nigeria my experience with infertility mirrored theirs; I just lived in another country. She explains that of the various types of infertility "barrenness carried the highest stigma." According to the Yoruba culture I was barren. I had been married for ten years and I was not able to have a child.

I visited West Africa when my mother-in-law died in 2001. At that time I had been married for six years and when I landed at the airport I could feel the stigma, just like the unbearable heat. It seemed that every woman my age had children in tow; all I had was luggage. I had come back to Mother Africa with no fruit.

Every aunty, uncle and relative mentioned it as soon as they said hello. Some went so far as to express that I had denied my mother-in-law the opportunity of seeing her grandchildren before her death. My sister-in-law on the other hand had had a baby within the first two years of her marriage. I could feel the stigma. Tongues were wagging!

In Yoruba culture, marriage is a huge celebration and is not taken lightly. It is the blending of two whole families, not just the husband and wife. Both families look forward to the culmination of their relationship and bond with the birth of a child.

As soon as I got married, my mother and mother-in-law culturally became sisters; they formed a very strong bond and became parents to both Victor and me. This also applied to our fathers and other relatives.

A Yoruba wife (whether she was born on African shores or aboard) who is barren is considered cursed. She is as good as being unmarried. She has no voice or value. People believe that if there are no children it is easy for the relationship to break up, as there are no blood ties. The birth of a child says to both families that they are now related by blood and those blood ties run deep. Not being able to have children in the Yoruba culture was and still is considered abnormal, it is a gross interruption in the natural order of things. The primary concern is the continuation of the family lineage. The pressure on the couple is immense. In some African circles it has led to many a family becoming polygamous, where the introduction of another wife is deemed necessary in order to have offspring. This is devastating to say the least, but that's a topic for another book.

It does not matter how far from the African continent you travel or live or were born, this cultural perception, and the pressure it brings is alive and well. Parents and grandparents take on infertility as a personal failure. Never before have I seen such a conflict between education and culture, trust me education doesn't win.

It seemed tolerable when I was in Canada but it was difficult whenever I went back to the UK or to Nigeria. I got looks of pity from my Nigerian relatives and a barrage of comments and questions and in some cases, blatant rudeness. Right from the beginning my parents-in-law were very worried; in fact they began worrying within the first few years of us getting married. Every letter they wrote made it clear they wanted a grandchild. That was their "yours sincerely" at the end of every letter.

Thankfully I didn't have pressure from my father; sadly he died within six months of my getting married. My mother on the other hand was a completely different story!

I know it was because she cared. She wanted grandchildren. She grew up in that culture though she had immigrated to the UK before I was born. My mother had all four of her children within five years. She had no idea of what my world was like. I didn't want to worry her; I could not tell her about the difficult time we were having trying to conceive. She was already going through other things; this would have broken her.

She kept telling me that members of her Nigerian community thought she had done something wrong or that I was cursed. She seemed to believe that I was intentionally trying not to have a child. In her mind, the idea of me not wanting kids, if that was the case, was preposterous! Life was marriage, then kids!

There was a time that the pressure coming from her was so intense I actually asked her to stop calling me because our conversations always ended up with her saying something that would set me off. It was so bad that on one occasion I asked her which bridge she wanted me to jump off. I had just about had enough. We were both under pressure but I could not take any more. I think she got the message.

After that, we had fewer conversations and they were much tamer. My understanding of the culture is not as deep as my mom's, so I can only imagine what she was going through too. She lives in the UK and travels back to Nigeria often. She had to deal with all the comments and gossips on the Nigerian front, which was no small feat because those people don't hold back. Believe me when I say, cultural ties are tough and traditional beliefs are extremely difficult to break.

My mom remains my number one fan and I hers. Regardless of her cultural position, she stood by me and with me and prayed for me. She never gave up. She was relentless in her faith that she would have grandchildren. Without her I would not be where I am today.

It would be unfair if I didn't say that the culture is really well-intentioned, but it ramps up the pressure on a couple to the nth degree and has been the cause of many a broken marriage.

I was blessed to marry Victor. Though he has the same heritage and upbringing as mine, he stood as a wall between me and all the madness. He protected me from hearing so much negativity. Our home was my safe haven because Victor made it safe for me. He made sure that all the insensitivity and nasty comments stayed outside our front door. He refused to succumb to any of the pressure. He made it abundantly clear that there was absolutely no pressure coming from him. He wanted children but as he said to me, he didn't marry me for that reason. There were so many ways to have a family and he was willing to explore all the options that I was comfortable with. In the meantime we sponsored children in Guatemala, Vietnam, New York and Uganda. To this day we still have children that we sponsor. It's a privilege to be able to make a difference in the life of a child. I never saw Victor's faith, or face flinch even once. I truly married an amazing man when I married him.

I am actually not aware of any culture or ethnicity that treats infertility kindly. There is certainly a little more understanding in the West due to education, but not in all circles. The misconceptions of the causes are rife and ignorance is alive and well in many parts of the world. My heart goes out to families who have this additional cultural factor. Doctors often suggested I de-stress my life to try and get pregnant. They had no idea of the pressure I was under. How do you explain the cultural conundrum in a ten-minute doctor's appointment? Having faced the diagnosis of infertility from three cultural perspectives, Canadian, British and Nigerian, I get it, and I understand the extent to which it can be isolating. Did it change my position? No. It just set another angle to the kind of crazy I had to be.

Round THREE

When it is dark enough you can see the stars.

– Ralph Waldo Emerson

I have always had fun buying a vehicle. You think your new car is unique. In my case it was a little bright red Pontiac Sunfire. It was a few years old but new to me. I thought it was fabulous; it matched my personality — RED! I had not seen that model before... until I drove it off the lot. Within two minutes I began to see Sunfires everywhere, especially red ones. It was the same with the diagnosis. After I learned about mine I began to meet women in my community who were either going through infertility, or had come through it. It was surprising how many there were. The infertility rates in Manitoba are alarming. The global stats had not changed much over the last few decades, but in Manitoba it was about one in five. One in five couples are infertile. That is one couple in every five houses down my street was living with what we were. The stats don't mean much unless you are one of them, and we were.

In my quest to find great stories I came across the bible story of Hannah. OMG! As the story goes, Peninnah was Hannah's husband's second wife and rival. Penninah had many children and she provoked Hannah, taunted her cruelly, rubbed it in and never let her forget that she was childless. It's one thing to be childless but to be taunted by another woman daily and have a pregnant belly right in your face, not once or twice but five times was too much to bear. After enduring what she did, I am surprised Hannah wasn't up on either a murder charge or assault! At least I was going through this in a more encouraging environment. If I were Hannah I am not sure that I would have kept it together. The good news is Hannah did keep it together and ended up having six children, me next!

Thirty days after the nursery was ready, I was pumped. But after three hundred days, there were a few discouraging moments; still, I blatantly refused to give in. Giving up was not an option. The stories and testimonials I read fuelled my dreams and encouraged my soul. It made the waiting easier. I read a story every day. There were times my very own mind told me I was crazy! Yep! I spoke right back to it. I talked to myself in my car all the time. Many a locker room chat has taken place in my car. Had I lost my reasonable mind? Yep! I had to fight my mind, my body and challenge my self-talk. Common sense and reason would advise me to accept the cards I was dealt. Crazy says take the cards and change the game. Then play to win! No excuses. As my friend says, an excuse is a skin of a reason stuffed with a lie. The craziness had already begun, why stop now?

One year went by and nothing happened. I still opened the

door to the nursery every day and I could see myself in there with my baby. My imagination was colourful and I fed it! Winnie the Pooh and I became closely acquainted. I bought stuffed toys of the whole crew — Eeyore, Piglet and Tigger.

Another six months, five hundred and forty-seven days in total went by and still nothing. I had planned a trip to Toronto one weekend when I got a phone call from my pastor asking me to sing at a church event. It was a Mother's Day event. I felt awkward and I was tempted to offer an excuse; after all I did have a plane ticket booked. How would I feel singing to celebrate the moms in our congregation and community when I so desperately wanted to be one of them?

I had to change my thinking and refuse to see it that way. I chose to see it as an opportunity to encourage moms. There was no doubt my pain was deep but I agreed to do it. I wanted what they had. I cried at home but I wanted to be where they were so I did what I knew I had to do. I would celebrate them by bringing my A game. I prepared to sing India Arie's "Eyes of the Heart." It's from the movie *Radio*. (I watched the movie again as I was writing this piece. It touches my heart every time.) The movie is a true story about an eighteen-year-old mentally disabled African-American student, James Robert Kennedy of T. L. Hanna High School in South Carolina, nicknamed "Radio." He is befriended by the school football coach and ends up becoming the coach's loyal assistant. He fights racism and overcomes many odds, learns to read and becomes a special part of the football team, and eventually he is accepted by the other students. Mine was not a physical disability: it was an invisible yet visible disability. I was disabled in the area of having children. It is something you live with every day. Every child's cry or giggle is a constant reminder... and I discovered there are children everywhere. Watching the movie, I was struck by Radio's persistence. He was constant, consistent and he challenged my heart and soul. This biopic by Michael Tollin helped me see that a disability does not need to handicap anyone. Radio did not allow his disability to define him. I watched an interview with James Robert "Radio" Kennedy many years after the movie. He still has a joie de vivre.

It was while on a ski vacation in Aspen, Colorado in 1996, director and producer Michael Tollin had picked up an issue of *Sports Illustrated* and read Gary Smith's article on James Robert Kennedy (Radio) entitled "Someone to Lean On." It was what inspired him to obtain the rights and begin work on a film version. He said perhaps what encouraged him most was his previous work with intellectually disabled people. In 1990, he had led a group of twelve Special Olympians on a trek up Mt. Kilimanjaro, and through the expedition, he came to fully realize the remarkable potential of such individuals. What I learned changed me: I could see that it was also possible for people dealing with infertility to climb their mountain if they were persistent and remained persistent.

That Sunday morning I took a deep breath and gave it everything I had. I sang to celebrate all moms, I sang for those of us who believed we could be moms, and for those who had given up; there were so many emotions. There's a part in the Radio movie where the school football team, "the yellow jackets," come running out on to the field with Radio in the lead... I felt just like that as I sang. No tears, just pride. I felt honoured. In my pain, with my disability, I sang my heart out. When I finished singing there was a huge ovation. My pastor prayed for all the moms and those of us who wanted to be moms and in that moment something clicked. I can't explain it but there and then deep down inside my faith and hope were ignited in a different way.

It had been a year and a half and our nursery was still bright yellow. It had all the trappings of a beautiful baby space — lovely, but empty.

I tried to be as healthy as I could. I remember making only one real lifestyle change. I was a huge coffee drinker at the time; I drank way too much coffee. I backed off and then gave it up completely.

Another year passed and still nothing. I was pregnant in my heart, so the longer I waited the more expectant I became. Every day I was getting closer to the dream. The waiting did not tire me — it made me stronger. Every day I woke up and went to that yellow room. After two and a half years I decided to go back to the doctor and get retested. We walked into the clinic and asked to be retested. Our doctor did not see the point, but he humoured us. So we took tests to see if anything had changed. It would take a few weeks for the test results to come back. A few weeks seemed like forever, but against the backdrop of already waiting thirty months, it was nothing. We sat down for the results. I could see that our doctor had some news; he was half smiling. I knew that whatever it was, it had to be good news.

He asked me what I had been doing. I said praying, dreaming in yellow and not drinking coffee. He announced that my FSH (follicle stimulating hormone) levels had dropped from 13 to 9. I was stunned, excited, floored. FSH levels don't drop; they only get higher with age. To get pregnant, your FSH levels have to be below 10. People can pooh-pooh my craziness but they can't deny my results. My doctor had no explanation. So what did this mean? He went on to explain that the results put us in a position where in vitro fertilization treatment was now an option. Yay! He then swiftly added that because of my age and medical history we had a ninety-five percent chance of failure. I'll be honest — I was elated regardless. All I heard was a five percent success rate! It must have been all that yellow paint. We had beaten most of the odds already—we were back in his office talking about an opportunity to get pregnant. We had already won!

From NEVER to a five percent chance! I can't begin to explain the elation. Granted, there were many hurdles yet to clear but now we had a chance. The previous year we were not even allowed to fly to the country where the mountain was let alone climb it. I gathered all my mountain-climbing gear with all the zeal possible. We knew that it was a journey with some steep terrain. We had no idea what lay ahead, but when you have nothing to lose you go all in!

Round FOUR

Hope is the little voice you hear whisper 'maybe' when it seems the entire world is shouting 'no'.

– Unknown

It was crazy, literally... In the in vitro fertilization treatment process there was so much to take in, the paperwork, the tests, the medication and the counselling. I felt like I was trying to take a sip from a fire hose! It was overwhelming, but we had a shot at getting pregnant so we were excited and committed.

It reminds me of the game shot in many Chicago Bulls games. Ten seconds left on the clock. Michael Jordan is dribbling down the court after an unfortunate turnover, all eyes are on him, everyone holding their breath and he gets an opportunity once the layup is made, he gives it everything he has got, he lands the shot and sheer pandemonium breaks out. We were on our way to the hoop — we were going to take the shot!

I got educated, I gathered as much preliminary information as possible.

We attended a few information sessions to learn more about the IVF process in the evenings as Victor had since found employment and was working during the day; it was odd to see all the people in the room. We were put in batches of ten or fifteen couples. Everyone in the room had one thing in common; none of us could get pregnant by ourselves. It was easy to feel a little awkward, but I was hopeful about the technology available to help us. There were a lot of tense faces, but I kept my hope buttons switched on. I had come a long way; I had come too far to give up now.

One thing was abundantly clear from the start — it was not going to be cheap. The in vitro fertilization process was expensive. So Victor and I scraped up all our savings and accepted that there were going to be two things on our menu for a while, beans and rice or rice and beans for many months to come. The sacrifice was worth it.

Around that time, coincidentally, the human resources department at Victor's company made some critical changes to their policies and benefits. The impact for us and other employees going through infertility was phenomenal. The changes meant that $5000 worth of fertility medications would be covered once in the lifetime of an employee that needs it. I could not have been more grateful. Some of the injections were $300 each so we were very grateful for the extra help. The rest of the funds needed were all we had left. There would not be one dollar remaining!

We paid the fertility clinic fees and started with counselling; they had to be sure we were suitable and stable enough socially, emotionally and mentally to look after what could be multiple children. We had no family, no relatives in Manitoba but we had a great church and a good circle of friends. They were our family; we knew if we needed help they would be there.

Daily injections were part of the process. I am not a fan of injections but I had to learn how to inject myself in the stomach... It had to be at the same time every day. I could not be five minutes late. I set the alarm on my phone to go off at 3:55 p.m. daily so I could inject myself at 4:00 p.m. One day I was driving down the street and I lost track of time. The alarm on my phone went off and I was right in the middle of traffic. I remember literally swinging my vehicle to the side of the road and pulling down my pants and stabbing myself in the stomach... I could see the driver in the truck next to me. You can imagine the sight. Unzipped pants, blue flowered undies, bare stomach and more, injection in hand then I stabbed myself. He was in shock . . . his mouth fell open . . . poor guy. He must have thought I was on drugs! I was, legal ones. Hey, when you want a baby that badly there is *no* shame. When you want a dream that badly you don't care, you do what you have to do!

The difference between a wannabe mama and bulldog is none!

The injections continued for a month or so and then there was one weekend when I overdosed the medication. I accidentally gave myself too much; I was frantic! Thankfully the pharmacist assured me that all was well. By the time I had taken all the medication, my stomach was black and purple. I had a lot of bruising and it was painful to look at and painful to touch. I had no space left to give myself another injection. We went back for more tests as they had several more things to check, more drama...

Round FIVE

There will be a few times in your life when all your instincts will tell you to do something, something that defies logic, upsets your plans and may seem crazy to others. When that happens you do it. Listen to your instincts and ignore everything else. Ignore logic, ignore the odds, ignore the complications and just go for it.

– Judith McNaught

Treatment seemed to last for an eternity. We finally got through it. We had set dates to return to the clinic. One of the doctors made his examinations and looked at the test results. I could feel something was a bit off when he sat me down. He had bad news for me; these were his exact words: "After the amount of medication you have had, normal women produce thirty follicles. In thirty follicles we usually find one or two eggs. You have produced only two follicles." He told me that the odds against me were so high that there were virtually zero chances of finding any eggs in my follicles. He asked me to abandon the process. Unfortunately, Victor had to go to work that day so I was there by myself. I was facing a very well respected physician who had my test results in front of him and he was asking me to go home. These were my exact words to him: "When I first came to this clinic a few years ago, you said I didn't even qualify for the desert, much less the Promised Land. I have come this far and I can see the Promised Land. It's not clear. It's blurry. But I can see it and you want me to go home now? NO!"

He asked me if I wanted to call my husband, hoping that Victor would talk some sense into me, and I refused to. I knew what his answer would be, he would tell me to stay put — I had lost my mind on this issue a long time ago and I was not going to be reasonable now. I could see the frustration on the doctor's face. He was getting redder by the minute and could not talk me into leaving. He tried the financial angle mentioning again the fact that the dollar meter would be running into the thousands if we made the decision to operate and check the two follicles we had. There was no question in my mind. The money was not an issue; we had put everything we had on the table, and we were willing to give it all. And I was done with everyone giving me bad news. I asked him "How do you want this? Visa, MasterCard or cash?" Now I was getting upset. I didn't know this doctor from a hole in the wall — who was he to tell me about what to decide and how to spend my money? He had no idea who I was and where I was coming from...

I called for my primary care physician who calmed me down. I learned from him that my chances were even less than zero. I guess they both figured I was really serious about not leaving. They agreed to go ahead and operate.

They harvested the two follicles we had and guess what? There was one egg in each one! Yay! A total miracle and they were grade A. (I had no idea that human eggs were graded from A-E, A being the best). Someone had egg on his face, no pun intended. The eggs were harvested and then Victor's sperm was collected to fertilize the eggs. I had heard "test tube baby" my whole life, it turns out that the eggs are fertilized in a petri dish. I guess "petri dish baby" doesn't sound that cool.

We came back a few days later for the final procedure to insert the fertilized eggs into my uterus. They inserted both eggs and the waiting began to see if they would stay in my uterus. The journey so far had been hard but I had my faith, family and friends to lean on. I barely breathed the next few days. I had to be careful and that was difficult. "With bated breath" — I now know what that means. Several days later I went in for another test; I gave a urine sample and left. The nurses advised me to call back in a few days for the results and they would tell me if we were pregnant or not. They wanted me to find a comfortable place and have a friend with me because they did not want me alone when receiving the news, good or bad. I went to Marcia's house; she had given me her keys as she had to go to work. My good friend Kim was with me. We were both nervous, we talked about anything we could just to get my mind off things and then the phone rang...

Round SIX

What you get by achieving your goals is not as important as what you become by achieving your goals.

– Zig Ziglar

I picked up the phone, it was the clinic. Kim looked at my face for an indication of the answer. I sat down. It was quiet, I waited for the words…it was a yes. We were pregnant with twins! Kim started screaming. It was crazy — she was so excited — a combination of hope, joy, and happiness all mixed into excitement. She was screaming so loudly I couldn't hear what the nurse was saying. I thought the neighbours were going to call the police. I actually had to call the nurse back. She understood — she was happy for us too. The clinic nurses had been on this journey with us from day one, they understood. I was in a surreal zone. It was so unreal, this twelve-year journey... Despite all the odds and all the many obstacles we had faced, we had finally won! I experienced so many emotions, all the disappointments, cultural issues and tears; we took the shot and scored.

The next part of the journey had begun and it felt like a dream, all the waiting, all the dreaming, all the hoping. It was finally here. It was a sobering moment. I had challenged life and won. I had fought a long, arduous fight, not without its scars or bruises, literally, but here I was; I was dirty, bloodied with a few broken bones but there was no denying, my opponent was down. I was on top of the world. Yes! Once we had calmed down I was speechless, and in awe of God. It was a true OMG moment. I felt a combination of relief, happiness, and fulfillment all at the same time. I cried. This crazy journey that had been filled with so much stress was now a thing of the past. I called Victor... there were no words... we were finally pregnant. My husband is not an overly expressive man but this was different. This got to him. He was quieter than usual. It must have been a mixture of shock and awe.

I had been dreaming of twins for years. My hope was for identical twin boys, I had bought clothes for twin boys. I knew our twins were fraternal because two separate eggs had been fertilized, but at this point I didn't mind — I was just happy to be pregnant. The clinic gave us ultrasound pictures of the twins, they were only a few days old, they looked like two little cells but I now had physical proof of my babies. I resisted the temptation to tell the whole world, a tough call but it was necessary. I wanted to spread the news but I also wanted to relish the secret for a while. I never thought I would say this, but I was thankful that at the time I got pregnant I was overweight so no one could really tell I was pregnant; that became a hiding place for me. I felt the fewer people who knew the better. I felt safe.

A friend of mine was confused; he thought we should be shouting it from the rooftops. I quietly explained in our culture we celebrate birth not conception. It's not for the runner who enters the race but for him who gets to the finish line; then and only then do the people cheer and the medals come out. When was the last time we gave medals to racers who just showed up to race? I love how Eric Thomas puts it: "Only execution is worshipped." I had no idea at the time how taking this position would protect me later on.

The next day was my first official day of being pregnant. I don't think I slept — I was so excited! My husband began to treat me like an egg, just about drove me crazy. I had to try and be a little more understanding, these were his babies too! I didn't know what to do with myself. Everything seemed fine for the first few weeks. Yes, I was glowing and very happy, and now opening the nursery door every morning had a brand new meaning. I knew this day would come. We were on our way.

I was required to take certain medications daily. I hated them because they smelled so foul but I had no choice. Within a few weeks morning sickness kicked in. It was awful! I have a natural aversion to vomit and here I was, heaving every two minutes. It was debilitating. I would literally wake up and go straight to the toilet and hug the bowl. My husband did not know how to comfort me. I was jealous that he could leave the house. I was between jobs and because I was really sick I would not have been able to go to work anyway. I struggled to get into the shower. There were days when I just sat next to the shower; I was so weak from vomiting I could not even get in. I couldn't move. Just prior to getting pregnant we had renovated our home and I had found this absolutely beautiful Moroccan tile that we installed in the kitchen and bathroom. Loved it! Good thing because I saw it a lot — up close and personal. It was my only companion for many months. To this day if I happen to see it at Home Depot, it brings back horrible memories. And there are still certain foods today that I can't eat because they remind me of how ill I was. Every day was a vomiting fest. It was so bad there were days when I was vomiting blood. My brain just couldn't take it anymore. I got to the point where I thought I was done — no more pain! I wanted to get off this train. I didn't want to be pregnant anymore. It was just too hard; I didn't think I had it in me to continue, but it was too late. These children I had longed for, prayed for, cried for, for years, I was now ready to give up. I was physically and emotionally spent. I was in so much discomfort that I was now ready to give in, give up on my dream. Pain can push you to that point. I held on but only just. I had heard all the stories of morning sickness and I thought that what I was going through was normal. I complained to the doctor. He prescribed a drug that made me feel even worse. My friends suggested ginger so I tried ginger in every form possible, no joy. I tried other over-the-counter drugs with minimal success. Nothing seemed to help.

The nausea was overwhelming and I became irritated easily. Certain smells drove me up the wall — white rice, raw chicken — and the only thing that tasted good was snow. I put trays on my deck and collected snow. It tasted good. It was the only thing I could eat without vomiting. I was fragile.

Thankfully all the ultrasounds were fine. I literally dragged myself to them with the help of a few friends. One day after a few months of this madness I heard a knock on the door.

I don't know how I found the strength but I crawled to the door. It was Marcia. She was shocked at how pale I looked; I could see from her reaction that I must have looked bad. She immediately bundled me into her car — no time to get shoes — and we went straight to the nearest Hospital. I don't recall all the details but within minutes I was in a hospital bed with an IV stuck in my arm. Thirty-four IVs later I could actually think. It turned out that I had hyperemesis, the same thing Kate Middleton suffered from in her pregnancy. It was like morning sickness on steroids! I was in a fog, everything was happening around me. I was very tired and my stomach was tender. I was transferred to another hospital where an ultrasound was ordered to check on the babies. I got to the ultrasound room, tired but relieved to not be vomiting as much. I lay on the table and the technician put the cold gel on my tummy and began to check on the babies and after a few minutes he said, "There is one heartbeat." I sat up immediately. I was confused. I asked, "Where is the other one? There must be a mistake." He checked again and confirmed, there was only ONE heartbeat. I lay on the table, cold, practically naked and broken, had I not suffered enough? One of the babies was gone. My twin, my baby…

My husband came in the evening to see me, we both looked at each other, we had no words…

My baby that I had waited years for… my baby that I had only weeks to meet was gone… What was worse was this time there was no response. Death was death. Life was pushing me to my very limit. I literally curled up in the fetal position but there were no tears. I was numb.

I didn't know what to say; I was hurt beyond anything I could imagine, but I kept my mouth shut. I didn't say anything I didn't believe. I let the tears that eventually came speak for me. I thought I would have to go through a procedure to remove the baby, but they said it was not necessary and that my body would expel or absorb it. My hospital room was semi-private so I had a roommate. She was young, about twenty-six. She was on kid number five; three different baby dads. She didn't really care. Wonderful. Our stories could not have been more different. Did I say life was unfair? I cried and I mourned for the little one that would never be. Thankfully I had only confided in a few friends so my grief had not become local gossip fodder. I was able to mourn and grieve in private.

Round SEVEN

Success is not measured by what you accomplish, but by the opposition you have encountered and the courage with which you have maintained the struggle against overwhelming odds.

– Orison Swett Marden

A week after we left the hospital I was still raw and coping as best I could when I bumped into a friend, who said something that jarred me from the fog I was in. She said, "You need to look up, you still have one baby left, fight for the one that is left." I was so blinded by my pain that I was only looking at what I had lost, not at what I still had. I still had one baby left. It was a light bulb moment and a switch in my head flipped. That thing that rises up when your back is against the wall and you fight like crazy with all that you have, that thing that makes a mama lion fight for and defend her cub. I got it! Something changed inside and there was now "crazy" in my walk and in my stance; from that point on, I had my fists up permanently ready for a showdown at any time. I was in fight mode, otherwise known as *beast mode*. I was ready to pay whatever price was necessary, even the ultimate one to protect the baby we had left.

I got up — in every way — and I began to feel better physically and to everyone's shock and horror I began job hunting. My friends had said no one would give a pregnant woman a job, not in the second trimester. Well, where there is a will there is a way. I became fearless. Guess what? I got a job interview with one of the largest registered charities in the province. I recall reminding the CEO three times during the interview that I was very pregnant. I wanted to make sure that he realized I would be gone in a few months. It did not faze him at all. He offered me the job as Grant Writer. I couldn't thank him enough. I needed to be focused on other things and to help others. I worked at the largest homeless shelter in this part of the country. My job involved writing grant applications for all of the programs that were offered at the shelter. I got to meet homeless people and I discovered how much I didn't know about them. I fell in love with them and I realized that the human condition is sometimes smelly, messy and painful but it does not negate humanity. Every day that I went to work I was grateful. Then there were those days when I would get lovely comments about my hair or clothing from our clients who had nothing. I was now visibly pregnant. They were as excited about the baby as I was. My baby became their baby. I often thought they were looking after us! They gave me perspective, daily. I was happy focusing on something else, and the paycheque didn't hurt either. I ended up finding a true purpose there and I was excited to get to work every day. I absolutely loved it! It was also a great distraction from the challenges of the pregnancy.

I felt truly alive when I was working so I worked to the limit. I witnessed compassion; the milk of human kindness lives in all people regardless of their situation. I recall a time when it was –40°C; our parking lot was across the street from the shelter and I was waddling from my car, feeling ten months pregnant, I was tired and my belly was huge. Some homeless people were lined up outside the shelter waiting to get in. It was brutally cold, yet they were concerned about my getting across the street safely. Once I was on their side I was still vulnerable to slipping on the ice but they ensured I got into the building safely while they still stood out in the cold. They were amazing people; always kind to me. I am truly thankful. I will always look after them.

I worked my tail off; I arrived early and left late. I loved my job. During that time the smell of turkey or chicken nauseated me. Can you imagine how I felt when two hundred turkeys were donated to the shelter for Christmas? There were some trying times but the nausea was worth the sense of fulfillment I found in my work. I was so immersed that my boss kept reminding me not to make a mistake and come to work on the way to the hospital when I was going to have the baby! I still chuckle about that.

I began to feel much better. I had to attend all the ultrasound appointments by myself as Victor worked out of town, so I recorded the baby sounds on my Dictaphone (I didn't have an iPhone then), and I wanted to frame all the ultrasound cards. I was pumped to be having regular ultrasounds. All of them after the second trimester were good. It was magical to be able to see the baby grow and move on the screen. At the final visit with my OB/GYN she said she was concerned about me going into premature labour, something I could not afford. I had been advised that that would have fatal results. My uterine lining was really thin after the operation to remove the fibroid tumour, so she decided to take the baby at thirty-two weeks. I had come this far; it was a very high-risk pregnancy and she advised it was safest, for my baby and me, to have an elected Caesarean section. She asked me to choose a date, a birth date for my baby. I had a few options to choose from and I chose February 5, the date I had immigrated to Canada — February 5, 2000. It held great meaning. Now my baby and I would have an anniversary in common.

Everything was all set. My family had flown in from the UK the last week of January 2007 so my house was full. On the morning of February 5, my three siblings, my mom, my husband and I bundled ourselves into my little van and set out for the hospital in the cold. I remember my brother Tim asking what possessed us to live in such a cold climate. It was freezing! Before they came they had joked about Winnipeg not being *that* cold. But that week we had a cold snap, they became believers! With the wind chill it was –52°.

I waved as we drove past my office at about 6:00 a.m.; we arrived at the hospital before 7:00 a.m. What I had hoped for and dreamed of seemed like it was finally coming true. Was I really going to get my happily ever after?

We registered at the desk and were shown to my room. All the procedures were explained and before I knew it I was in the operating theatre. The nurses were lovely, and it didn't take long. I was given the spinal block and I was numb from the chest down; within minutes they began the incision. Just the fact that

I was in the operating room brought tears to my eyes; I spent the first few minutes asking myself if this was really me. I would have pinched myself but the spinal block had put my body to sleep. The doctors said I could watch and I was delighted to have a chance to see my baby being born. I had seen the procedure on television, but this time it was me... I looked in the overhead mirror (which my husband thought was so morbid), but I didn't come this far to take a back-seat view or watch from the sidelines; I wanted to be front and centre.

We had decided along the way not to learn the baby's sex until the birth because we were willing to accept a child of either sex; after the journey we had come through, a healthy baby was plenty. I did have a thing about twin boys but I had already accepted the fact that I was not having twins anymore — I was focused on what I did have. Did my heart ache for the twin I lost? I would be lying if I said it didn't. It's a pain that you learn to live with but that day the pain was drowned in the joy of seeing a new life being born. It was fascinating. I loved seeing the birth. I really didn't feel anything except some tugging. I saw them make the incision and then there was some tugging and pulling and within a few minutes they pulled out the baby.

Surprise! It was a girl! She was a lovely one too — 6 lbs. and 18 inches. I waited to hear her cry and she did. Her APGAR scores were 9. She had the biggest brown eyes...

Tears. Lots of tears, tears of joy! In just a few minutes I had gone from Vicki to Mom. My dreams were realized, my dreams had come true. It is hard to explain all the emotions.

Victor and I wanted to name our baby the way we were named in a traditional Nigerian naming ceremony eight days after birth but the hospital would not have released her without us registering her birth and giving her a name. At the beginning of the pregnancy we had spent a long time picking boys' names when we were hoping for twin boys; Michael had been a joint favourite, but we had not agreed on a name for a girl. So we chose a girl version of Michael, Michaela. It means: Who is like God? But we chose to spell it differently: Miqaela. Both Victor and I are avid scrabble players. So we tried to get the most points out of her name. Anyone who plays Scrabble knows that the "q" is worth ten points. We did not have any relatives living in Canada and we found that we were often in circles of our friends and their parents, some of whom were single so we "adopted" a few seniors. One of them was a lovely senior lady originally from El Salvador, Alicia. She became a part of our family and when we had our daughter she automatically became *abuela* which is Spanish for grandmother. She also chose to spell the name with a "q" It resonated with me so "q" it was. Miqaela. I know ... crazy huh? After winning this battle we could name our child whatever we wanted! We would give her other names at her naming ceremony eight days later.

I was so in awe of the miracle of her birth. I spent the better part of the day just staring at her. Life as I knew it, my status, the trajectory of life, everything had changed in that one moment. Hello happy ever after, it was crazy!

Round EIGHT

Sometimes the smallest things take up the most room in your heart.

– Winnie the Pooh

She was a beautiful baby, I was in awe of how she looked. She had huge brown eyes. I stared at her all the time, every minute. I couldn't believe how beautiful she was. I was also in shock at how my life had changed. It was so hard to sleep; I kept thinking it was a dream and if it was I didn't want to wake up. My family took tons of pictures. I remember my sister Liza saying, "You've done good sis, she is really beautiful." I couldn't believe that someone so beautiful was mine.

The euphoria of giving birth to a beautiful baby definitely masked the pain of the healing Caesarean incision — walking and sneezing were challenging. Thankfully it was in the same place as the myomectomy so just one scar, but I was not thinking of wearing a bikini any time soon, my stomach muscles were shot.

I remember having really pleasant nurses at the hospital. They took the baby so that I could sleep. Many nurses and doctors checked on me. They poked and prodded. Sometimes residents came around with the doctors. At times it was quite embarrassing. Since then, I have always maintained that after you have a baby all dignity is lost. These people were pure strangers to me, trainee doctors and nurses, many of them asking to look at my private areas. By the end of my hospital stay, I felt like asking the janitor if he wanted to have a look too. I was very tired. My natural adrenalin was slowly waning and exhaustion was kicking in. I really had not slept much. I could not breast-feed Miqaela as my milk had not come in yet and I was engorged. Her pediatrician came by and asked a few questions. He suggested that I was ready to leave the hospital. I don't know what came over me but I remember saying, "Doctor, if I cannot stay, tomorrow's headline will read, 'Patient kills Doctor'." I was joking but I don't think he felt that way. He told me to stay as long as I wanted! The hospital gave me formula for Miqaela, which I fed her using a tube attached to my finger. I had heard how a baby should be 100% breast-fed for the first six months but the first few days it just didn't happen for me. I had no milk for a while, but I did nurse her as soon as it came in. After four days, I was ready to go home. The weather outside was still so frightful even Jack Frost would have run away! There were serious weather warnings that morning. Skin would freeze in ten seconds. It was so cold the hospital staff would not let us leave the hospital until we had warmed up the car for thirty minutes. Her car seat was so completely covered in blankets; I was worried Miqaela might not be able to breathe!

My siblings kept saying that they could not believe how cold it was. My mom swore never to come back in winter. On the Sunday after the birth Victor and I went to church. My family all went to their various churches online. It was a funny sight, five laptops on my dining table. But we love our Manitoba — it means *Great Spirit*! It resonates with our life view. My family thought that living here was just another crazy decision we made in 2000. It's not the place of choice for many, but we are pioneers by nature. Breaking ground in new places is part of our DNA. There were times when we thought we were crazy to try and succeed in Winnipeg, but we are not ones to back down from a challenge. If we did uncommon things we would get uncommon results. We now had uncommon results.

We got home from the hospital, we were all very excited, remember that Winnie the Pooh nursery? Now after three long years I got to put my baby in my own crib. It was a long wait but when it actually happened, it didn't feel like it had been that long. I finally got to physically do what my heart and mind had done many times over in my imagination. The next morning I was on my way to the basement to have some quiet time, which for me is praying and meditating. My husband was concerned about me using the stairs because of the stitches I had. I reminded him that when I was dreaming of having the baby, I was always downstairs meditating and now that I had the baby I was not going to stop going there to pray and meditate, and just be grateful. My child meant the world to me but she didn't mean more than life itself; she had become part of our lives, not 'life' itself.

Life the way we had known it had changed drastically. I enjoyed being a new mom. I was ecstatically happy but drained and tired. It is hard to explain but every parent or caregiver knows what I mean. Now it was time to plan her traditional naming ceremony and dedication and we only had a few days to plan it.

Round NINE

A name represents identity a deep feeling and holds tremendous significance to its owner.

– Rachel Ingber

As soon as we got home we immediately began to prepare for Miqaela's Nigerian naming ceremony. We saw it as an opportunity to share our daughter in a special way. We had the gift of being part of three cultures. Our heritage is Nigerian, Victor and I were born British and had also become Canadians. We decided to blend the three cultures as best we could to create a ceremony that had meaning to us and all our friends and family that would be attending.

On the eighth day Yoruba children are named. We wanted to give our baby names according to the Yoruba custom. The ceremony is called an "*ikomo.*" It is not a baby shower albeit gifts are presented. It is where the parents officially name a child in the presence of family and friends. We had given her the names for her birth certificate so we could take her out of the hospital legally but now it was time to celebrate her and speak to her future with the names we were going to call her according to Nigerian custom.

Yorubas believe that a name is a special thing, a blessing and an indication of your destiny, a forecast into your future. It is not taken lightly. It is a treasure and an indication of your birth circumstance. Your name explains how you were born and we certainly had a story to tell.

We had decided to call her Miqaela, a female version of Michael which means: Who is like God? We believe that in giving her that name our daughter's life will be an answer to the question. Jordan was the name we picked for her second name. It has Hebrew origin meaning "one who descends" or "to flow down." We indeed believed that she descended from heaven to us, a blessing that flowed down to us. Both names sat well with us and what they represented was important to us. For her Nigerian name we chose the name *Oluwafemi* which simply means "God loves me". I felt that way. I felt loved. It was final. Miqaela Jordan Oluwafemi Olatundun.

We had asked a close Canadian friend to "send a name" also. It was quite a foreign concept to him. In our heritage it is believed that items of clothing will become old or toys will break and will one day be discarded or given away but a name will stay in the life of the child forever. It cannot get lost and it remains part of the child's history and destiny, it is a lifelong gift.

Her paternal great-grandmother who is still alive but very old and lives in Nigeria sent a name. At the time of her birth we had already lost Victor's parents so we asked Victor's auntie to send a name on their behalf. All in all she had seven names as gifts. As the ceremony began, the names and their meanings were presented first:

- *Miqaela*, Who is like God? (given by Victor and me)
- *Jordan*, To flow down. (given by Victor and me)
- *Oluwafemi,* God loves me. (given by Victor and me)
- *Opetosioluwa*, God is worthy of praise. (maternal grandmother)
- *Iretioluwa*, The hope of God. (paternal great-grandmother)
- *Ilerioluwa,* The promise of God. (paternal uncle)
- *Abeke*, We asked for her to care for her. (paternal great-grandmother)
- *Elizabeth*, My God is an oath. (maternal aunt)
- *Thera*, Untamed. (close Canadian friend)
- *Ifedapo*, Love blended together. (maternal great-aunt)
- *Ugochukwu*, God's Eagle. (maternal great-aunt)

We selected our friends to present traditional Yoruba birth gifts of water, honey, sugar, salt, a bible and we added music as a part of our Canadian and British culture. During the ceremony, our pastors who presided over the event prayed over the baby and us. Then he called for the gifts. The first person with a gift stood up and said, "I bring water" and then presented the gift of a bowl of water. The pastor with Miqaela in his arms then dipped his finger in the water and touched it to her lips and read out all the positive attributes of water and ascribed them to her.

"Just as water is used to wash things clean, so will your life be, it will bring cleanliness to all things it touches, just like water is used to bring many to safety so your life will bring safety to many people around you" and so on and so forth. He went through all the presentations in a similar way but when it came to music we had a friend sing a special song for her. We believe that just as music is soothing, encouraging and makes people happy, her life will be the same to all those around her.

Then we had cake and refreshments and celebrated. My brother Tim and sister Lola were the masters of ceremony; they made us laugh a lot.

It was an awesome ceremony; it was great to be able to blend our friends, family and all three cultures. I recall coming home with Miqaela and receiving all the phone calls and congratulatory messages and best wishes. The recurring theme from my Nigerian aunties was that we should try and have some more children, and quickly. I couldn't believe it. I knew they meant well, but I thought, I've just had one child, a complete miracle, yet the hungry culture wanted to get its own five cents in; I didn't let the pressure get to me. Of course, there were the underlying tones of "you should have a son to continue your husband's name." I refused to play the game. A child was a child whether it was an only one or not and was special regardless of its sex.

The fertility clinic had told us if we wanted more children we would need to go through the whole process again as we did not have enough eggs to cryopreserve some, but I was done. I could not go through what we had just been through again. I was happy with being the mom of one child; we didn't have any more savings anyway. Our family was now complete. I was beginning to get into the groove of things and just when I thought life had calmed down, then drama…

Round TEN

You never know how strong you are until being strong is the only choice you have.

– Anonymous

It was early in May 2007, I had gone to the hospital to see Miqaela's pediatrician so that she could get her first immunizations. She was nine weeks old. It was a normal day, nothing out of the ordinary. We had gone early, about 9:00 a.m. We arrived at the clinic and the immunizations were administered without a problem. On the way home traffic was particularly heavy. I felt quite small on the road in my little red two-door Pontiac Sunfire. There were lots of trailers around me, especially on the highway. My car didn't have all the proper latch hooks for a car seat but we found a way to make it work. It was like a mini Fort Knox in the back, Victor made sure. I was driving on the highway when I felt a clip by another vehicle behind my car and it began to swerve and in a bid to stop I pushed the pedal right the way down thinking it was the brake — it was the accelerator. The vehicle spun out of control and I T-boned a trailer. My whole life sped before me in a few seconds but at the same time it all seemed to happen in slow motion. When my little car came to a stop it was crushed, completely totalled and the air bags had deployed. My face was burned from the gunpowder in the air bags and a hole burned through my jacket in the chest area. I was in shock and very disoriented then horror set in; Miqaela was in the car and she was not making a sound. I hurriedly got out of the car. By this time, people were gathering around and by some miracle the police, the army and paramedics all happened to be in the area — they came running as soon as they realized there was a baby in the car. I recall an army officer grabbing the car seat from the car and asking me her name. He started calling her name. She was non-responsive. She was not moving. He could not tell if she was breathing. She was only nine weeks old. At this point I just about collapsed as my heart sank. The paramedics kicked into action and put us both in the ambulance. I became hysterical. How could this be happening to me? I sat in the ambulance with tears streaming down my face, and the only thought going through my head was that I had killed my baby. I phoned Victor but I could not reach him. So I called Marcia. She was making her way to the hospital. I called my church; one of our pastors was on the way. I was frightened, lonely and really low, I must have said a thousand prayers. It is so difficult to describe what that low felt like. The only thing I can think of that would remotely come close is jumping out of a plane with a parachute that would not deploy and you know that hitting the ground is going to be the eventual and inevitable end. They rushed Miqaela in and I sat and waited and waited. It was a long wait. I was falling real fast; I was pulling at the parachute chords frantically... nothing. My friend arrived and I broke down. My pastor came shortly after and prayed with me. I coasted in the air... I ripped at the chords... nothing... My thoughts were screaming... I had killed my child. I had already lost one baby. This could not be the end... after the twelve-year wait and finally having the dream, was it going to end in tragedy?

Even though I was distraught, something in my heart was not willing to accept it. I had to fight for her; I kept my thinking as positive as possible. I will be honest in saying that my faith levels were not high. I was hanging in there. I was hurting. My friend tried to comfort me. Then the doctor came and I stood up to face the challenge. I braced my heart... His face was stoic so I really couldn't tell what he was about to say. Everything was hazy, my palms were sweating, my knees were shaking and my heart was pounding. He said, "She's deeply asleep." He explained that because she had just had her immunization shots she was in a very deep sleep. At that point the parachute deployed and I had just enough time to avoid impact… I crumpled into the seats nearby and I started to cry out of sheer relief.

Round ELEVEN

Sometimes you have to do what's best for you and your life not what's best for everyone else.

– Unknown

As you might expect there was so much excitement when I first brought Miqaela home. Gradually I settled into a daily routine. I had regular visits from the public health nurse and on every visit she would ask me if I ever felt blue. I thought this was an odd question — at first, because I am quite a happy-go-lucky person. I felt fine up until my family left, but now I had to look after her by myself every day while the whole world went to work. I missed work. A lot of women find that hard to admit because society "says" that you should be all consumed with the new baby and happy to be at home with them. I found things to do... but I could swear the walls were getting an inch closer every day. I thought I might be getting a little depressed — postpartum depression maybe? I found activities, library reading groups for moms, tots sing-song groups, a new moms group, but it was not the same as going to work. Despite how I felt I tried to tough it out. I talked to lots of moms who could not understand why I missed work so much. I had taken my professional exams and become the Human Resource Manager at the shelter before I left on maternity leave. I found it very hard to make the adjustment from a high-pressure position to changing diapers and nursing a baby all day. I was exhausted all the time; my neat house was not as neat as I liked it any more. I loved being a mom and I loved working, why couldn't I have both?

I recall a friend who had been a top award-winning pharmaceutical rep for ten years. She was beautiful, sassy and I loved seeing her in her power suits and short spunky hairstyles. Then she decided to have a baby and unfortunately the bottom fell out! When I saw her six months after the baby, she looked terrible, she hated being at home and I could see she was very depressed. She told me that she missed work but couldn't go back because she had saved up over the last few years so that she could stay home with her children when she had them. It was tough to see her this way and then she had another child and just about died within herself. I was determined that would not happen to me. I understood that every situation is different and I was going to do what was right for me.

Salvation came by way of my maternity benefits coming to an abrupt end. I had only been working at the shelter for four months before I had Miqaela, so I didn't qualify for a full year's maternity leave. My employers had graciously given me seven months off work instead of the twelve weeks I should have had. I loved being a mom but I could not stay at home. I felt like the walls were closing in on me. I had to get out daily so I did what was right for me; I decided to go back to work when the leave was up. A big shout-out to women who stay home with their kids — they are amazing women — and a super shout-out to moms who home-school their kids, neither of which I can do. Thankfully I was courageous enough to admit it and not allow societal pressures to dictate what was right for me.

The only way it could work was if I could find suitable childcare for Miqaela. The additional income would be helpful as our expenses were increasing with all the baby supplies we needed. Finding childcare was a challenge, for an infant it was not only pricey but also very difficult to get. Putting her in the hands of strangers was a worry for me; I had heard many horror stories. A friend of ours was almost offended that I was going back to work; though he didn't say it, his attitude seemed to be, "How could you go back to work and leave her after all you have been through?" Simple answer: I didn't want to lose my job, I loved my daughter and I loved my work too, and I was passionate about both helping people and being a mom. I had to find a way to make it work.

It didn't take too long; after just a little searching, I was able to find a friend to look after my daughter. Sharon offered to care for Miqaela. Sharon was the friend incidentally who when we were going through our infertility situation had offered to be a surrogate if we needed one. It was very obvious that she loved Miqaela a lot and looked after her like she was one of her own — Miqaela literally had two families. I felt very comfortable with Sharon; she was the perfect caregiver for Miqaela and it put my mind at ease that Miqaela would be safe.

I returned to work at the homeless shelter. It was hectic, going back to work was also quite a transition but I managed as best I could. It wasn't easy but I came alive at work. If it wasn't for my friend looking after my daughter it would have been impossible because daycare spots were very hard to come by. In Manitoba you have to get yourself on a waiting list the minute the pregnancy stick turns pink! I believe that all workplaces whose employees are of child-bearing age should have a daycare available on site if possible. It would drastically reduce costs, absenteeism and the employees' stress and mental health issues. (I will get off my soapbox while I am ahead...)

I got into a routine of nursing Miqaela in the morning before I left for work. I expressed milk so Miqaela was fed predominantly breast milk. I believe that breast milk is best but I supplemented with formula and had no guilt about it. (I discovered everyone has an opinion about how you should feed your baby; again I did what was right for me.) My routine began as early as 4:00 a.m. I had to pack the baby bag with clothing for daycare, get myself ready for work and pack lunches. I then had to drive to Sharon's house and drop Miqaela off. I was always late for work but I always made it, sometimes through slow-moving traffic, always grateful to be there. I enjoyed working and I loved the challenge of making change happen as well as being an internal advocate for employees and an external one for homeless people, and a mommy too. Working for the homeless shelter, I always left work grateful because I heard people's life stories daily. My life paled in comparison to the hardship I saw some of our clients going through daily. We think that most homeless people are grown-ups but they are not always adults. The youngest homeless person I met at the shelter was fourteen days old. She was a beautiful little girl. It was very sad; there was no difference between this little girl and mine.

I am glad I was true to myself. I was happy to be back at work and I was gradually getting back into the flow of things. It satisfied my passion to help others and the lawyer part of my brain. Being a former attorney, I really enjoyed advocacy and every now and then I did have occasion to go to court on behalf of homeless people as a social justice advocate — I love a good fight! That's why I became a lawyer in the first place. After work, I was able to completely switch off and become a full-time, fully engaged mom. I was excited to pick up Miqaela and play with her. I was happy. I could enjoy the best of both worlds.

Along the way there were many happy occasions where I could bring Miqaela to work for some staff kids events where I got to share her with my colleagues. There were great days like my first Mother's Day that I enjoyed celebrating at work for staff and the clients. But I will never forget my first Mother's Day at church. As soon as I heard my pastor say "Good Morning, happy Mother's Day," I lost it. I cried the whole service. I did not hear one word. I was overwhelmed with the idea that the trajectory of my life had changed so much. This little girl had literally changed my world. I was happy after waiting so long, and then getting to see this miracle... Wow! I was still going over in my mind how incredible the last few months had been when I heard my pastor say "Amen." The service was over. Sometimes it takes a while for reality to sink in but on that day it really did. Now I was one of those moms I sang to a few years earlier. I was a mom for real and nothing was taking it back.

I knew that Victor wanted more children but the thought of going into major debt to make this happen was something that we could not handle. My body could not take another bashing like it had, let alone my mind. So we settled on having one child and life was good. I was working and happy. He completely understood how I felt; he had been through it with me. We gradually started to rebuild our lives and our savings, and get into a routine. Then as usual life came knocking…

Round TWELVE

The moments of happiness we enjoy take us by surprise; it is not that we seize them but that they seize us.

– Ashley Montagu

My first Christmas as a mom was fantastic; Miqaela had her first picture taken with Santa and life was good. My friends had been such amazing supports since I had her. Marcia, Kim and I had had a really busy and exhilarating year so we decided to treat ourselves to a spa day and an overnight stay at a nice hotel at Christmastime. We arrived at the hotel and in true girl fashion we talked about nothing and everything at the same time. We booked a suite at the Clarion Hotel and we spent the evening talking, eating and having fun. Miqaela was with her dad, and like every new mom I called a hundred times to see if she was all right. But with the girls, it was like being teenagers all over again. We were being silly and goofy and having a good time. I started telling the girls that I didn't remember when I last had a period. They say it takes a while for things in that department to get back to normal after baby. Both girls looked at each other and then at me and they started giggling. They both shouted "You're Pregnant!"

It was the furthest thing from my mind. My daughter was barely ten months old. I knew what being pregnant was like — I assured them that I was so not pregnant. I had not been sick, so I was very sure.

The girls kept giggling; they asked me to get a pregnancy test from the drugstore and just to humour them I got three. There was a very faint pink line on the first test, it was unclear, inconclusive, plus I was feeling amazing; being pregnant for me means being terribly ill. I was ecstatically happy, life was good and I was gradually getting back to my pre-baby self. So we ordered food and continued to have fun. Then I took another test, and there was a very faint pink line again. It was still not very clear but they were convinced I was pregnant. I thought they were being silly.

The only real way to find out was to go back to the clinic. I had to go anyway as I had been told that the fibroid tumour I had would begin growing again after I stopped nursing. I stopped nursing Miqaela in November. The earliest I could get into the clinic was January 2008.

In January I went in to check on the state of the tumour. After the ultrasound and examination, they confirmed that the tumour was not growing and had not grown throughout my pregnancy — phew! But something else was growing... I thought maybe a polyp or maybe adhesions. I waited to see the ultrasound pictures of what the doctor said was wrong with me. Then he announced "You're pregnant." I think even he was in shock as he gave me the ultrasound picture of a seven-week-old fetus. I really was pregnant again, and this time it was free! This time we were not even trying as they say. We got pregnant all by ourselves. Crazy.

I had fought life and won and now it was handing over the goods! I didn't know what to do with myself. I was shocked. Our doctor gave me a big hug; now we would be that story of hope that he told to the next couple. This time my pregnancy was absolutely fabulous! No morning sickness whatsoever, I didn't so much as sneeze. I felt amazing the whole time. It was the extreme opposite of the first time. I was still considered to be high-risk so I went through all the standard tests, but I refused an amniocentesis; the results would not change my position. My doctor was concerned because at my age there was more risk the baby would have Down syndrome. I carefully explained to my OB/GYN, it would not make a difference to us. A child was a child — Down syndrome or not. Also, there was an inherent risk of complications if the baby were pricked with the needle used to collect the sample of amniotic fluid. I wasn't having it. I didn't want to take what in my mind was an unnecessary risk.

I was asked if I wanted to learn the sex of the child, I refused again. Baby number two! In my heart I thought a boy would be nice as I already had a girl but I didn't mind. I was looking forward to just having a healthy baby. I was open to nature's surprise. This time it would be different. I would get a full-term paid maternity leave for one year! I could make up for time I missed with Miqaela.

It was a textbook pregnancy with no morning sickness. I went shopping often, I loved work, I volunteered. I felt on top of the world! I really understood why some women love being pregnant. I felt pretty, big but pretty. It was just plain fun.

Early one very cold winter morning when I was about four months pregnant, I was taking Miqaela to Sharon's, driving on the perimeter highway going 40k in a 100k zone. The road was slick and slippery. The perimeter highway was notorious for being like a skating rink on such mornings. As I was driving I hit black ice, what happened next was insane. I spun out of control so badly that I crossed over the median into oncoming traffic. I was facing a semi-trailer head on. He saw me and swerved to miss me. The white car behind him I hit head on! I was driving a new Chevrolet Venture at the time; it was a complete write-off. Thankfully there were no fatalities. I had minor visible injuries but I was scared for the baby I was carrying, and Miqaela who was sitting behind me; she was startled and started screaming. The most important thing was to ensure that Miqaela and the baby I was carrying were OK. I had some whiplash from the accident; I could already feel it. Luckily a Good Samaritan driver stopped a minute later so that we could be warm until help arrived. We made her late for work but she saved us from the freezing temperatures. Thank you stranger!

I eventually managed to get my daughter to Sharon's only for her to announce that she was ill and could no longer look after Miqaela starting immediately. I didn't know what to do. I called another friend and she offered to care for my daughter for a few days while we found a minder for her. I literally had to drive 40 km away in the opposite direction from work and back, and then drive to work and get there before 8:00 a.m. When it rains it pours! We struggled to find care. Luckily a friend of a friend knew someone near my office. She turned out to be an amazing caregiver for my daughter. She treated Miqaela just like one of her own children.

In the middle of all this there was some good news, I saw the doctor as soon as possible after the accident and learned that the baby was OK. Phew! I could breathe a little and it wouldn't be too long after that we would be seeing the new baby.

Round THIRTEEN

It's not the mountain we conquer but ourselves.

– Edmund Hilary

Despite the fact that this baby had been naturally conceived I faced the same risks with this birth that I did with Miqaela's. The lining of my uterus was still paper-thin. I was asked to pick a birth date again. My OB/GYN informed me that they would be taking the baby at eight months again to avoid my going into labour. July 31, 2008 was the date I chose from the options I was given.

Everyone in the office was convinced that I would have another daughter. They said I was "carrying low." My colleagues had even bet on it.

My obstetrician knew we would have been happy to have a son. In fact she joked that she would put her fingers in between the baby's legs if it was a girl, just to make me think it was a boy. D-day came; it was another elected Caesarean section. They began the incision, Victor who is squeamish, was uncomfortable, I could only feel a little tugging and then out the baby came and the doctor said, "It's a boy." I didn't believe her. She had to bring him over and show me his genitals. I had a little boy, he had a great cry and I was so overcome, a boy, yay!

I had another decision to make while on the operating table. My OB/GYN had raised the issue of a tubal ligation in one of my prenatal appointments. Victor and I could not come to common ground so I told her that I would make the decision after I had the baby. My doctor felt that as I was already open and on the operating table it was the best time to do a tubal ligation, if we wanted to. She gently reminded us that we had been very lucky. We had been through two very high-risk pregnancies with no casualties. She didn't want to see me again, in the best possible way. She said I was at risk of having adhesions. I agreed to a tubal ligation. It was absolutely the right decision for us. We did not want any more biological children, but I have to say that even though it was the right thing, somewhere in my heart I still mourned that I would not be able to experience the birth of a child again.

I remember there was a code pink alert in the hospital after I had the baby, someone had picked up a child and walked out of the hospital. This was a high-alert lockdown. I slept with Michael on my chest. I could not fathom someone stealing him. Thankfully they were able to find the baby. The nurses were checking on me every two hours, so sleep was impossible and the food was designed to send you home. We gratefully left two days later. We took our son home. Baby number two...and almost forty-one years old; I was done. I had made my contribution to humanity. No more babies for me! I was happy and yet a little sad. A few weeks after the birth, I met up with my friends Marcia and Kim and mourned the loss. I would no longer be able to have another child. In my case the operation was irreversible. I can't explain why I was sad. I had not anticipated that I would feel the loss so deeply. I think my heart mourned because it was so final. Logically the decision made sense. I was in my forties and I had a daughter and a son. I would be endangering my life by having another child, yet my heart cried as I said goodbye to that part of my life. It helped to be with my friends to officially acknowledge it and mourn. It is hard to explain...closing that door hurt but I made my peace with it.

Once again I was in heaven, baby heaven. He was a cute little boy, he was very active and he had a loud cry. We had a tough go of breast-feeding. He was just shy of six lbs. We called him Michael. There was no question about it. It was a name that was so significant to us in so many respects. Victor had always wanted one of his kids to have the initials M.J. — his nickname during his basketball days (Michael Jordan). The name Jordan was already taken by Miqaela so we called him Michael Jonathan. Now we had two "M.J.s"

Eight days after his birth we planned his *ikomo*, his traditional naming ceremony. Relatives and close friends were also asked to bring names to celebrate his life and future. We chose the same gifts as we did for his sister. We had planned a simple but sweet ceremony. Then life checked in to see if we were still breathing.

I had been home a day or two when the public health nurse came by to check on me, but I was on my way to the mall. I was excited and happy and I had forgotten she was coming.

I was already at the front door; Michael was in the car seat. Miqaela was with her Godmother; I wanted to get out to some sunshine. The nurse was insistent; I grudgingly agreed to go back in the house. She said it would only take a few minutes. She took my blood pressure and asked me to lie down immediately. I was confused. She took it again and said we needed to call an ambulance. Why? She explained that my blood pressure was so high that I was in the stroke zone; she needed me to get to the hospital straight away. I felt great, but I now know that that's not a true measure of health. She explained that is why they call it the silent killer. I was taken aback. How could I be facing a stroke? Life again! If there is one thing I had learned, life can, and will strike at any moment, but I had made up my mind to fight back every single time. Victor was due home shortly so I waited for him and he took me to the hospital. They kept me on a ward; they were desperately trying to bring my blood pressure down. There was no explanation; all I was told was that blood pressure could spike after childbirth.

Meanwhile, I was planning the naming ceremony; people were flying in from other countries for it. I explained these things to the hospital staff. They agreed to give me a day pass to leave the hospital, but at my own risk, and I had to report back at 10:00 p.m. I was grateful. The ceremony was amazing! My mom and sisters came from the UK and others were there from far and wide. I explained to our guests that I had to leave because I was due back at the hospital. I was running late and the hospital called me to come back. I stayed in the hospital for five days. They were eventually able to bring down my blood pressure and get it under control. Recovery from this birth was easier as I had been down the path before. They usually give you a ten-week recovery after a C-section but I pushed the limits a bit. The pain was brutal but I healed quickly and was driving six days later. Not advisable, but I had no choice as Victor had to go back to work three days after the birth.

I got into a routine with the children. I made the most of my maternity leave. I did as many special things as I could with them. We made lots of memories. It was busy and exhausting at times but I didn't let any of the tiredness bother me; I reminded myself daily what it was like to be childless. This always put things in perspective quickly. I enjoyed every smile, every giggle and every poopy diaper! I pinched myself once in a while, just to check that this was really happening to me. I was literally living my dream.

After many serious slips, falls, nail-biting moments and loss I finally reached the summit of the mountain. The climb was filled with danger at every turn. I have lots of emotional, mental and physical scars as proof but I also have a huge sense of achievement daily that drives my passion and purpose on a crazy level! Yes, there were days when I didn't think I would make it but I just kept reaching for one slippery ledge after another.

The higher I climbed the more the sounds and voices of those that said it was impossible were fading. Crazy is really what gives birth to the impossible. I attempted the climb knowing that according to the experts I only had a five percent chance of success. Yet there I was at the summit, tired and exhausted but there nonetheless.

There is nothing that can describe the feeling at the top.

Nothing.

My children are now seven and nine years old; watching them grow has been fascinating. Seeing them strive for their own dreams is rewarding, but teaching them to be crazy in their pursuit of life is my favourite part. Every time I hear them say "mom" I am reminded that fighting for the dream was worth it. Fight for your dreams; don't let anything or anyone stop you. You know what you want and why. Go after it with everything you have, giving up is not an option. Life doesn't usually fight you for what you have now because you already have it. Life fights you for a future that you could have if you are willing to pay the price and persist until you get it. Don't ever back off, back down, turn off, turn down, shut off or shut down your dream no matter how long it takes. Be reminded that along the way people will tell you that you are crazy and they will have evidence to prove it. But for you "NO" is not an option. Go and get what belongs to you.

When people want to remember that they have been somewhere they record it in some shape or form, they take pictures, make movies, carve their initials in trees, spray graffiti on walls, or write on something with a permanent marker. The view at the summit was amazing; absolutely breathtaking; the only thing left to do was record it. I chose to inscribe in indelible ink on a rock at the summit; this book is that inscription. Unleash your crazy and win!

Part TWO

Introduction

The people who are crazy enough to think they can change the world are the ones who do.

- Steve Jobs

I guess this is where most people would end the book, but you have read my story so you know me by now. This should logically be its end but there is nothing logical about crazy. Welcome to the other side of my journey. Common sense says to accept the cards you have been dealt, but crazy takes the cards, changes the game and plays to win. In my pursuit to have a family, I blatantly refused to accept the status quo or common sense; not only did I change the game, I changed the rules, then I played to win and won. I learned so much about myself and what it takes to win. In fact I became a completely different person in the process. I unleashed what I call "my crazy" and I changed my life forever. This part of the book is my invitation to you to not only find your crazy but also unleash it and use it to change the world.

Incidentally, I just got back from a gymnastics competition; Miqaela was awarded a bronze medal. I cried, not because she didn't get the gold. I cried because I realized that my crazy continues to pay off. It has been nine years since I had her and even though I get dividends every day from just watching her grow, this one was special. I would never have had this moment if I had settled for common sense and not become crazy enough to fight to have her and Michael.

Now I know how to harness all the pain and pressure and make it into a tangible form. In the beginning I thought the whole experience was about having a family, but in the process I have learned how much power I have and how to ignite it; now I live with more passion, more power and more crazy in all areas of my life.

I once heard one of my favourite motivational speakers Eric Thomas say, "Don't waste your pain." Today I have not only used my pain, I have analyzed it, employed it and obtained business success with it and beyond.

In this second part of the book I describe the principles I learned during my fight against infertility, and how I was able to use these principles to achieve business success. It is a different concept to combine a story about fighting infertility and business success principles into one book, because they don't seem likely partners. I didn't think so either, but my experience proved different. They have a lot more in common than you would think.

I have discovered that principles are principles and they work in every arena, be it looking for a baby or looking for success in corporate or non-profit enterprises. I hear crazy ideas all the time and I never want to be one of those poor souls who says an idea is stupid and crazy and not at least hear it out. Tim Westgren says and I agree, "Don't be shy about believing in your ideas – even if folks around you think you're crazy." The principles that I share can be used in any part of life. I say start by first setting your crazy free. We are all designed with it. It is part of our DNA and we are all what I call POA (Pregnant On Arrival). We are all born with a dream and the crazy ability to fulfill it. Often that potential is not nurtured or encouraged and it can become dormant or die if you let it. The good news is that it can be awakened and unleashed. It is never too late.

I recently read about a young graduate from Florida State University, who wanted to make her butt look better in white pants so she cut the legs off of her pantyhose. She must have looked amazing because she went on to create a new undergarment. She scraped up all her savings, $5000 that she earned selling fax machines door-to-door for two years, and implored manufacturers to make a prototype. Everyone thought it was a crazy idea. She began cold calling buyers. The rest they say is billion-dollar history. Hello Sara Blakely of Spanx. As of 2015, Sara Blakely was worth $1.06 billion USD. It's a phenomenal story, what grabs me the most is her crazy. Crazy is what gives birth to the impossible. It also takes guts and courage to take a risk.

How about a local British Reggae musician who sold Jamaican jerk chicken at the Notting Hill Carnival once a year and turned chicken sauce into a multi-million-dollar enterprise. Welcome Levi Roots of Reggae Reggae Sauce.

Who would have thought it possible to put in our pockets more power than it took to put the first man on the moon?

Crazy idea? Yes, but the world changed, didn't it? Now we have iPhones, iPads, iPods, i-everything. Thank you Steve Jobs.

The list of crazy entrepreneurs is endless — Jeff Bezos, Founder and CEO of Amazon; Reid Hoffman, Co-founder of LinkedIn; Larry Ellison, Co-founder and CEO of Oracle Corporation; Jack Ma, Founder and Executive Chairman of Alibaba; Richard Branson of Virgin; Mark Zuckerberg of Facebook are just the very tiny tip of the iceberg of crazy success.

Let's not forget extraordinary visionaries and founders of non-profit organizations and registered charities who have employed their crazy and impacted the world socially on an unprecedented level. I call them non-profit entrepreneurs. Myron Reed, William Ryan, William Friedman, Dean Hart and Frances Jacobs of United Way; Scott Stahl, Frank Shankwitz and Linda Bergandahl-Pauling of Make-A-Wish Foundation; Robert Pierce of World Vision International; Paul P. Harris of Rotary International; John van Hengal of Feeding America; Craig and Marc Kielburger, Founders of WE day; and the list goes on.

The one simple thing they all have in common is that at one time or another, someone said their ideas were crazy. They disagreed and went for it anyway. It is obvious that crazy is a prerequisite for success, it's an absolute must. We now applaud their craziness, which has become our new normal. I see parallels between fighting infertility and attaining success in business as a non-profit entrepreneur because I have lived through it and have proven success in both. My period of infertility is a constant reminder that I can turn any situation around and win despite the odds, and I believe it is a framework for my business success and life in general.

My scars have become a source of inspiration. My pain has become my power, my persistence — my path and my passion — my mission. What might have broken me has become a true source of strength. Every time I face an obstacle I relive my story and reconnect with my "why" and the way forward becomes clear again. I mentally walk through my battles and revisit the victories, and revisit the stories of others who have gone before me; this shoots adrenalin into my soul and revives my crazy fighting spirit. I hear the word "mom" when my kids wake up and the crazy in me arises. My hope is that this part of the book will do the same for you too.

As a visionary, I am naturally one of those "why not" people. I don't just think outside the box, I break the box, redesign it and build a boat and think a hundred miles outside of that! That's how I got my nickname The Girl Noah (TGN). I see opportunities to build "Arks" everywhere. According to the MacArthur Study Bible commentary, Noah "takes a hundred years to build an unsinkable gigantic box big enough to accommodate a volume of 1.4 million cubic feet equal to the capacity of 522 standard railroad boxcars." He does so before the world had ever seen rain. This is not only an outside of the box thinker, but a crazy thinker, my kind of crazy. I admire the Noah story; there is just something about it that resonates with me at a core level. I heard he built the Ark in his backyard and didn't he have the last laugh? Can you imagine what the neighbours were saying? Today he would have been sectioned off or declared crazy. The story of the Ark is depicted really well in the movie, *Evan Almighty* — just plain funny, but it makes my point. As for then filling it with animals, I rest my case. Robin Sharma says, "Every visionary was reviled before they were revered and ridiculed before they were respected."

As a visionary and risk taker, I can't always wait for all the pieces to fall into place, in fact all the pieces are rarely ever in place. It takes crazy to still believe that things can happen despite the odds and I don't ever want to be cured of my craziness. I can only imagine how much better and innovative our world would be if everyone set their crazy free. Our combined crazy could become the future generation's normal. If we don't take those risks then we deny them the opportunity to create a better, stronger and more phenomenal world. I actually trust in my crazy ideas and believe that I can change the world. My advice: crazy is the new money, get you some.

I have wanted to write a book about business success principles in language that everyone can relate to for a while. I just didn't know that infertility would be my platform. I am a voracious reader and the books that have had the most impact on me have been ones with simple principles and clear concepts that I can use immediately. Everyone who heard my idea of combining business with infertility gave me that "this is crazy look." This part of the journey is written in a very simple format describing the principles I have learned from my experience and how I successfully applied them. They can be applied to any project — business, non-profit, NGOs or life itself. Do they challenge the status quo? Yes. Are they simple and easy to understand? Yes. Are they crazy and a little out there? Uh huh! Did they work? Read on. Enjoy the read as you learn the principles to help you unleash your crazy!

The Girl Noah roars!

Perspective

Surviving failure makes you bold, out of devastating failure comes spectacular events.

– Linda Gottlieb

It all started in January 2010. My children were now three and a half and two years old respectively and life was busy but good. I worked full time and I loved my job at the homeless shelter. But I had been there for four years and though I was very dedicated, I had become bored. It felt like there was nowhere for my career to go. I was the Human Resource Manager and I had ascended as far as possible. It felt like there was a lid over my head and I needed a challenge of some kind. I discussed this with my team leader and when a position running the medical clinic at the shelter suddenly became available the management team asked me to take the job. I did not have a clue how to run a medical clinic.

The challenge was just what I needed. I figured that administration was administration, whether it was the clinic or the shelter. It was a change and I had to grow and learn new skills; I loved that. My team leader gave me plenty of support and I worked hard and learned a lot. The administration of the medical clinic required that I gain some basic medical knowledge and terminology. I went after knowledge and advice. I took a few courses at a local college and I gained a few friends in the medical field. I became hungry to make a huge success of the clinic. I enjoyed creating organizational firsts — opening the first eye clinic for the homeless in Canada, and in conjunction with a local university the first dental implant program for homeless people, as well as the first gym specifically for them, which all led to lots of press and media coverage. It was fun helping to bring change and attention to the lives and conditions of so many people that society had forgotten. I felt really fulfilled every day. I had a sense of purpose; I drove myself hard and set the bar high.

As with all good things, they come to an end. I spent two years establishing an amazing clinic only to find myself back at the same spot. There was nowhere else to advance. There was nothing else to add to the clinic. I had a staff of forty volunteer medical professionals — doctors, chiropractors, dentists and optometrists to name a few, all of whom had my utmost respect. I worked with some of the best professionals in our province. Nothing else could be added and the Noah in me became restless. My pioneer heart was uneasy.

It was January of 2012 and I could sense that life was about to change. It was one of those nigglies, a gut feeling or something; I just wasn't sure how the change was coming. I could feel life's breath on the back of my neck so I knew that it was not far off.

In the meantime the commute to work was becoming more challenging; increasing traffic made it more difficult to pick up the children from daycare on time. I lived over an hour away from work and the journey was hazardous in winter when the roads were icy. It was stressful but I felt that it was a small price to pay for a career I loved. Most of the working population hate what they do for a living. I was an exception. My sense of purpose is measured by lives touched or changed. I am a causal human. I made a difference every day I went to work; I was truly satisfied and fulfilled. Then one day, out of the blue, I got a call from the executive director; I didn't think anything of it. I knew I had recently made an error, which I thought would mean a meeting with my team leader and a slap on the wrist, but unfortunately, that error cost me my job. I was in shock; I felt betrayed. I had dedicated six years of my life to the shelter; I had worked really hard and now it was all gone. It hurt! It felt like such a loss, I felt drained and it seemed like a disaster. But life happens. It had been a good job and I loved it; I had been stuck but I was comfortable. With hindsight I realize that it was not really comfort — it was a rut and you know what they say about ruts. Laurence J. Peter aptly describes a rut as "a grave with the ends knocked out." It was sad but more shocking than anything else.

On the drive home that day my mind was going in many different directions; what was going to happen next? It was going to depend on the way I saw this crisis and how I responded to it. Life happens to everyone; what matters are our responses. Did I cry? Yes, it was my human way to express pain. I hurt because I was going to miss the people I served and the relationships I had built. It was like a divorce, a death. I had to acknowledge the mistake I had made and forgive myself first. As a human, I am flawed. It was easy to blame others but the leader in me couldn't do it. I took personal responsibility and even though it was painful, I also chose to forgive the wrongs I felt were done to me; it was a costly lesson learned. I know that holding on to unforgiveness is like drinking poison and expecting the other person to die, so I made a conscious decision to move on and not hold any offence. Easier said than done but I managed to pull it off.

I was facing the prospect of looking for a new job; I had not looked for a job in six years. I rediscovered that looking for a job is a job in itself. I had to revamp my resume and reinvent myself, and that was not all bad. It gave me a break in my routine and a chance to refresh my life.

There were a number of things I did that helped me gain a new perspective after losing my job. I consulted my NASCAR team, a core group of a few friends and family members I talk to when the bottom falls out. You know — the people you can call at 2 a.m. and even though you have not spoken to them in many months you know they will pick up the phone. When life happens, I talk to them to keep my head on straight. I had a flat tire, in fact a major blowout, and I needed a pit stop. When faced with a flat tire I have seen many people slit the other three tires and become depressed, rather than fix the one tire. I needed the one tire fixed and quickly! I called them all; every member of the team went to work on my behalf. Every one of them supported me, they all gave me some good advice and they all encouraged me to move on. My husband is on the team and he told me not to worry (he was one of those who got the 2 a.m. call as he was in another country at the time). I recall what he said: "You have lost nothing because wherever you go you take you with you." He reminded me of all the amazing things I was able to accomplish in the past six years. He felt I would do the same wherever I went.

It was then I realized that working at the shelter had been a training ground. If I had understood that earlier I would have paid better attention, I would have taken more notes. I had gone to a "street university" for six years and I didn't even know it, or at least I didn't think of it that way at the time. Everything I learned there was part of a journey and I began to look at all I had learned and gained rather than look at the things that had gone wrong. Once I changed my perspective I literally jumped up and down because I was excited about how much I had gained in such a short time. I had gone to "leadership and management school" in an unusual way and earned a "street MBA." I was more skilled, better equipped, more experienced. In appreciation, I actually sent my ex-team leader a thank you card for all the amazing training I had received. I left the pit stop with a completely different mindset.

First, I decided to clear my head and take a break. There is nothing like a holiday to help with perspective. Just before I left for the break I applied for a job. I was surfing the Internet casually one evening and found a job opening for an executive director. From the job description I knew I could do it even though it had a big title. It was a big drop in pay but the challenge of leading a team was more exciting. I applied and landed an interview. It was a good interview but I was very bold — I had been through enough in my career that I cut to the chase. I made my position very clear. My exact words were: "If you do not want change please do not hire me. I am a change agent. I don't want to waste your time and I don't want you to waste mine. I will be taking a huge drop in my salary expectations to take the position so I am here because I want to be." There was no time to be politically correct, integrity was more important. I wanted them to know what they were getting. I was not at all sure they would offer me the position. I cannot imagine what they were thinking; at least they had thirty-two others to choose from.

Directly following the interview, I boarded a plane for the UK to visit my sister Liza, who also happens to be on my NASCAR team. She encouraged the fresh perspective, fresh start and new hope. While I was there, I got a call offering me the job. I guess they heard me and decided to offer me the position. Being honest has its rewards. I thought, what a twist of events... I had left the shelter as a manager and here I was the new executive director of a non-profit organization, all within twenty-three days; it was a whole new world!

I decided this time around things were going to be different. Pain was a great teacher! I was brutally honest with myself. I now had a fresh perspective. No job was for life! I knew that when I began the new job I had to plan my exit from day one. It's a strange thing to say, but I say it in the most positive way. I had to have a strategy for how and when to leave, what my legacy would be and then I would work backwards from there. On day one, as per Stephen Covey, I started with the end in mind; I began planning an exit strategy as soon as I arrived.

At the shelter, I had devoted so much of myself to the cause that often both my family and I took a back seat to my job — not anymore. Over the six years some of my identity had become wrapped up in my job. I drew the line in the sand early this time; who I was and what I did were two very distinct things. This time I was happy to give my all, but even "my all" had boundaries and balance. Knowing that no job lasted forever was freeing. Gone were the tunnel vision and deceptive thinking; I reset my priorities. I still had battle wounds from the last war and the lessons were still fresh. For me, my faith and family come first. They had kept me sane through the last battle and will always be there for me in the future.

It's crazy to say to yourself on the first day of a new job, "When will I be leaving and how do I want to leave?" but it's a perspective that will serve you well. I would rather make the choice than have it made for me. I usually put in place a three to five year plan and give myself an option to review and renew at the end of the first five years. This approach has kept me accountable, challenged and safe. It is a tough position to take; it is definitely not for the faint hearted. I usually set the bar for myself very high. I believe you determine where you want to go and you set a time limit. The clock starts ticking on day one.

Pregnant

Every birth comes out of labour pains. The most difficult task is not about being pregnant with visions; it's about delivering an impact that inspires lives.

– Israelmore Ayivor

After I got back from holidays, I set out to discover what I had got myself into with the new job. It was a great cause! I am a causal human — a natural born advocate, so anything that requires any kind of advocacy gets my attention. My training as an attorney was always helpful. It was called Anna's House, named after Steinbach's first female physician, Anna Schilstra, who specialized in obstetrics in the early1900s. At the time, the organization was built around the Canadian Prenatal Nutrition Program and looked after low-income families by providing some family resource services.

As soon as I arrived, I could tell immediately that staff morale was low; they had lost their team leader four months before. The centre was located inside an RV Sales Park in a dingy looking place. It reminded me of the old English workhouse for the poor, like in *Oliver Twist.* It felt hidden away; no one in the community knew where we were or what we did.

I thought about how ironic it was for me to land at a non-profit organization that advocates for kids and families. One thing that helps me keep my cutting edge is my ability to remind myself what it was like to not have a family. I never want to forget what it was like to be childless. It remains a mental tattoo for me to this day. I hold the family unit in high regard and because children are so small, often invisible and inaudible, they bring out the advocate in me, and here I was in a job where I would spend every day as an advocate for children and their families.

In my quest to find out about this organization I talked to community stakeholders. As I introduced myself they always looked confused. They often asked what our organization did. It was almost embarrassing. It seemed like I had gone from working for one of the most well-known shelters in our region to this place on some planet in outer space; from a several-million-dollar operation to an organization that was struggling to pay for essential resources. I had no idea what I had let myself in for. My annual budget for the clinic at the shelter was more than the annual budget for this entire organization. I was fascinated with all the organization did but no one in the community knew anything about us and there was no funding to help communicate this.

Anna's House is located in Steinbach, Manitoba, a very wealthy and generous community. It is a faith-based community located in southeastern Manitoba. Visible poverty and homelessness are rare. One would think that financial and in kind support would come easily to the centre, but that was far from the truth. I soon learned that the community had no idea what we did because we didn't tell them. If they didn't know about us they could not help.

I mentioned earlier in the book that we are all POA (Pregnant on Arrival). Every human on the planet is born with the capacity to dream; we are all pregnant with that ability, but what we do with it is a personal choice. I am a dreamer. I knew the first thing I needed to do was to get pregnant — pregnant with a vision. I talked to my staff team to learn about them and learn their thoughts and opinions. My chats revealed that they had witnessed many organizational miscarriages and abortions. I learned that every director before me had promised that they would move into a new facility, but didn't deliver, though not for lack of trying. Funding constraints are the plague all non-profit organizations have to deal with and they did not want any more disappointment; they did not want to be pregnant anymore. Too many times the stick had turned a positive pink only to end up in a miscarriage or abortion. The last few years had been challenging for them. When your dreams have been dashed often enough, you stop dreaming. I got it.

The first few months I spent learning to understand where we were from the inside and dreaming about where we could go. I could already see "Arks." I could see them everywhere. I had inherited a lot of things that needed sorting but I still set aside the time to dream. I had my eye on something. I created a mental picture of where I saw us going. My staff didn't care and

I understood, but I wanted to court them and get them to see what I could see. I wanted to take them "out on a date" but I had to build a relationship first. It would take a while for them to make eye contact, let alone "go out on a date." My staff had been there done that and had heard it all before. They gave me that "so who the hell do you think you are" look; they were tired. When I explained my background I could see their eyes glaze over. They just did their jobs, which were not very highly paid.

I have to share a huge pet peeve; there are some amazing non-profit organizations out there doing some amazing work, but they spend their time scrounging for money to be able to keep their doors open. Sometimes they literally have to beg. Why? It can be exhausting. That is NOT good! (My soapbox moment…)

I could sense compassion fatigue. I understood that my team was tired. They liked the work but they did not feel they were heard or seen. How do you get a disillusioned and hurt staff to come out on a date? I needed a quick win to peak their interest. I had to make the first date impressive. It was time to dust the cobwebs off my dating skills. The good thing was that I had an entire female staff so I could understand, to some extent, the things that they would enjoy. Most women have a nesting instinct; we like to make where we live look amazing and homey. I figured that my staff spent more of their waking time at work than they did at home but where we worked was not pretty. It was not inviting. So I decided to give our building a facelift to make it more attractive. We had a small area in the back corner of our building called the Clothing Depot; it was a blah space. No, blah is kind, it was downright ugly! The public donated clothing and toys in black garbage bags and old boxes. We put them in the back just like that. If we had time we did some sorting, if not then they remained in the bags. Moms would come in and if they needed anything they would rummage through the bags and take what they wanted.

One day, I was in our kitchen getting my lunch near the Clothing Depot and I saw a young mom come in. She started rummaging through the garbage bags for clothing for her newborn and my heart broke. I don't cry easily but I could feel the tears stinging the back of my eyes. How could we put a new mom through such indignity? I couldn't stand it. We were supposed to be helping. We didn't have much to give but respect is free, we could give respect to our participants. I shut the Clothing Depot down that day. You should have seen the look of horror on my staff's faces. We had always had a Clothing Depot, that's the way we had always done it. They were upset. They were not happy with me. I was the bad guy. I had brought in my city-slick ways and they were not having it. That "date" idea was slowly fading with every passing minute. If I asked them on a date they were going to flat out refuse.

They say it is lonely at the top. It's true but I was not budging. What was right was right. I approached the board about sprucing up the building a little and they saw my point, but there was no money to do anything. The savings we had were earmarked for a new building and it was not a large amount. I had to find a creative way to get it done.

Following the meeting with the board, I began to look for philanthropic service organizations like the Rotary Club, the Lions Club and other generous private organizations. I was familiar with the Rotary Club, so I raised the idea of going to them for funding; both the board and staff explained that they had been there done that and were unsuccessful. I was undeterred. I explained that I had not been there on our behalf and I was determined to get different results. I called the local president and in effect invited myself to one of their meetings. He agreed. I thought of putting together a neat PowerPoint presentation but opted for going with my heart. I took my speech with me, literally.

I arrived a few minutes early. I wore a very bright red jean jacket and I had my hair in dreadlock braids. Bearing in mind I was deep in Mennonite country, it was like arriving at an Amish settlement in punk rocker gear with spiky gelled hair. My entrance was memorable, put it that way. I stuck out, that was the point. I arrived fully loaded! With lunch and all the niceties out of the way, I began my presentation. I had brought a bunch of the black garbage bags filled with clothing and I put them in the middle of the floor; that was my presentation. I explained what our organization did and how in our bid to help moms we were robbing them of their dignity. I invited them to pick an item for one of their children or grandchildren. Not one of them took me up on the offer. There was silence. They were mortified this could be happening in their community. They wrote me a cheque for $1000, which was what I requested. My first win! I had asked them to designate the cheque for the specific purpose of renovating the space, so they could rest assured the funds would be used for that purpose only. A thousand dollars is not a lot of money but in my world it was a fortune, more importantly I could use it for leverage and pull some favours and community support.

I asked a designer friend to help. I told her that we had a shoestring budget, so we would recycle, upcycle, do whatever had to be done! Thankfully she agreed. She was willing to help us create a small store. She ordered some slat wall, special hangers, a mannequin and paint. I mentioned it to the staff team. They were curious but still unimpressed. The area was taped off and work began undercover. It took about twelve weeks to complete. Then came the big reveal. My designer friend had created a beautiful store with a monochromatic grey colour scheme. It looked like a real little "boutique." We stocked gently used clothing for children ages 0-5 years old and some maternity clothes for expectant mothers. Beautiful was an understatement — the store looked like a little Baby Gap store. The difference was that our clothes were not for sale.

I was proud. This was the perfect date! I called in my staff team and showed them first. They couldn't believe it. They were in shock at how awesome the store looked; I could see they were happy and proud of it. You never really know how successful a date is until you hear about it from a third party. Well, it was all over the local news, it was in the paper, on the radio and our participants came in and were asking how much the clothes were. It was great to tell them the clothes were free. Dignity restored.

We have since renamed the store the more inviting "Clothing Café." Participants could grab a coffee from the kitchen and "shop" at the same time. Within a week of the store re-opening, I heard some of the staff team giving tours of our building and the highlight, of course, was the new store. It was a small victory but also a taste of things to come and I could sense they were slowly beginning to believe me. I continued to gain small wins each day and soon we were not just dating, we were in a full-blown relationship, an item. Their getting pregnant with vision was still a way off, but this was a good first step.

The most compelling reason for finding a new space for Anna's House was safety. We were located in an RV park on a major highway. We were difficult to find. (I remember being late for my job interview because I could not find the place). For the first few months in my job, I missed the turn off the highway driving past the centre many times because there was only a small window of opportunity to safely make the turn. I worried about being rear-ended. The moms who came to the centre faced the same dilemma every time they came. Then there was the added risk of young children being run over by the constant flow of traffic — people looking to buy an RV were not expecting children to come running out of our building. On more than two occasions we caught children by the seats of their pants running into the paths of trucks. Every time I heard our front door open I worried about a child getting hurt. I could not bear the thought of losing a child but it was only a matter of time; we were an accident waiting to happen.

When I asked why we were in this unsuitable location I was told that it was all we could afford at the time. We lost our previous premises because the property went up for sale and we could not afford to buy it.

A pregnant teen was on her way to see us one afternoon, driving a vehicle under the supervision of her guardian when she pulled into the parking lot and thought she was pressing the brake —instead, she pressed the accelerator and the car crashed into my office. It was quite a shock! Obviously my concern was for the young mom and baby but what was really scary was had one of our toddlers been outside as they usually were, it could have been a fatal accident. It was time to move.

I knew that if a child were ever killed, we would never recover as an organization and the community would hold us responsible. I made it my job to inform the local business community just how dangerous our location was; it was not apparent to the general public because of how hidden away we were. I could see where we could go, I was pregnant with the dream of a new facility and it was contagious. Vision is contagious. I have often referred to myself as an *imagineer* and a visionary. I cast vision. I draw big pictures and ask people to help me colour them in. I put that picture on my wall then I break it into small pieces. An art teacher once told me, "Take care of every square inch and the picture will take care of itself." I was taking it one square inch at a time.

After several months, I put a huge sheet of paper on one of our walls and called it "The Dream." I asked the staff team to write down things they would like to see in a new centre if money were no object. The sheet remained blank for a few weeks; then I began to see items slowly appear, before long the sheet was completely filled.

I started to cast vision with the team collectively. I gave them permission to dream about where we could go. I am not sure if they believed I could actually take them anywhere, or if they thought I was just plain crazy. I think probably the latter. They had been at the current location for seven years. I shared ideas, possibilities, and opportunities and they started to believe. The

Clothing Café was proof that we could have nice things. It was a preview of what was possible. I began to see creative things on the dream list — stroller parking, air conditioning, full accessibility. The list was getting longer and as my first date was impressive I could feel a change. After a few months of courting and a few more small wins, the stick finally turned pink, they got pregnant! They began to dream like me. Sweet!

Persevere

I believe everyone is pregnant with a dream. Some people end up with a miscarriage because they feed their doubts, fears, insecurities and the opinions of others.

– Mandela Dunamis

No one decides to get pregnant just for the sake of it. Couples who want children have no idea what their journey will be like or what it is going to take but they usually plan as best they can. They are given a due date once the pregnancy is confirmed and they hope for the best, but there are no guarantees. It was no different for us. At the centre, we were pregnant, but only just. I didn't make a pregnancy announcement or celebrate just yet. It was easy to think that we had reached a milestone, but I knew better; it was only the very beginning of our journey. It was the time to plan for the best, prepare for the worst and face the future and persist regardless of the obstacles that would come our way. I am an extremely positive person, an eternal optimist but I am also very practical and I knew it would have been naive to think that it was all going to be smooth sailing. The best advice I could give anyone embarking on such an uncertain journey, which is often the case in business, is to decide from the get go that quitting is not an option.

A few months into our first organizational trimester (ten months in real time), I was asked a very honest question by the longest-serving employee, Jocelyne, who had been at the centre for several years, an awesome family outreach worker, brilliant at what she did. She had seen three directors come and go, and the way she often looked at me told me she didn't think I was going to last. She asked me if I was really going to change anything else. In my enthusiasm I explained that I was going to turn the place downside up. I could see our potential, what we could be. I could see an Ark, a big Ark. I was going to radically change things — the "Clothing Café" was proof. Wrong answer.

I could tell Jocelyne was not impressed. She loved her job and wanted stability and here I was declaring that we were pregnant with a big dream. The next day she resigned. Boom! Jocelyne might as well have dropped a bomb. It was not good; it came out of left field but she had made her decision and explained that it was not a personal one against me. It is not normal to have a painful contraction in the first trimester. I broke the news to the team at our weekly staff meeting; they did not take it well. After that it seemed as if the others were also on the verge of leaving, or at least contemplating it, and I felt they were just barely hanging on. The whole team went into panic mode, their lovely little family that had been together a long time was being broken up because of me. The most stable member of the team was leaving and they were watching for my reaction. I did not let my feelings show, I was sad but I did not let panic set in. The new vision, the Clothing Café and the good things that had happened since I arrived didn't seem to matter on the backdrop of losing their trusted friend and colleague. I thought that the fact that we were pregnant with a big dream was enough to keep everyone on board and excited. Not true, I realized that this journey was going to have casualties, some early on, but I was not expecting a contraction at this time. I went into my office took a deep breath and relived some of the successful moments I had had; I used those victories as pre-natal vitamins and I took a healthy dose daily. I made up my mind there and then an abortion or miscarriage was out of the question no matter how many people left the organization. Loss or not we were going to carry this baby to term. As with many pregnancies, there are many things that you lose or give up — your body, your appearance for example. Friends have told me all kinds of things they gave up while they were pregnant. One of my friends had to give up all her cute shoes because her feet were so swollen, I recall losing teeth as my baby was leaching calcium from my bones. Loss of some kind was inevitable; I settled that in my mind and kept myself focused.

We had a goodbye party for Jocelyne to celebrate all that she had achieved and sent her off nicely. She was obviously aware of our dream to eventually move to a new building. As she was leaving she chuckled and said to me, "Call me when you get into the new building." It was one-third sneer; one-third "I dare you" and one-third "Really? No one has ever done it before and neither will you!" There was a glint in her eye. It wasn't a malicious remark; it was an out and out challenge. I wasn't upset in fact I was pumped! They were fighting words to the Girl Noah. I love a challenge and this was a massive dare. I was jumping up and down on the inside while trying to maintain a calm, collected exterior. She also gave me a parting gift, which I treasure to this day; a gorgeous vase with an inscription: *Good actions give strength to ourselves and inspire good actions in others. - Plato.* She had no idea that she had lit a match — no, she had ignited an inferno. I continued planning for a full-term pregnancy and safe delivery of our dream and as I hit each setback, I would make adjustments. I refused to quit. What I didn't know was the obstacles and losses were just beginning.

I used everything I knew to keep the vision in front of us. The team was experiencing a lot of change. They had just begun to dream with me and Jocelyne's departure was a huge loss, this was akin to spotting in the first few weeks of pregnancy. It was scary. In quick succession the next blow hit. The dietician who had been on staff for two years suddenly announced that she was also resigning to get married in China, a second casualty; it could not have come at a worse time. I could feel a miscarriage coming on... We were down two team members; there were only five of us left, we were bleeding. Thankfully, after much bedrest and reminding the team about our "why" things calmed down. I kept vision casting by painting pictures of what could be and things progressed slowly.

The last few months of the "first trimester" were tough as we weathered each loss. In the middle of those losses I hired two new team members. It was a good move because I set things up right from the interview stage; I had impregnated them with vision before they came on board so there were now three of us whose expectations were high and shared the same mindset. The new employees thought like me, they fit in nicely and the organization began to stabilize. Our internal environment had begun to change. I could feel the sense of expectation rising and I encouraged it every opportunity I had. It was still a little uncomfortable but we were putting one foot in front of the other as best as we could.

A few more months later, we were gradually getting comfortable and our pregnant belly was growing and showing. We carefully passed the first trimester, the initial danger zone. This is the point when most families announce their pregnancy. I was beginning to feel like we were gaining some weight but I was not comfortable enough to tell anyone outside the organization yet. Around that time, a gentleman walked in off the street and asked to see me. He introduced himself as Keith. He explained that he felt the need to give back to his community. He had been searching for what to do and came across our organization. Keith was not doing very much in the evenings. I asked him what he did for a living; he said he was a painter. I did not miss a beat. My staff team know that I am an opportunist — if the fruit is hanging low I will grab it and bite into it. I bit on this opportunity immediately and I asked if he could paint our space. I was shocked that he agreed. He not only came in to paint in the evenings, he brought reinforcements, his wife and son and other helpers came with him. Our space got a complete overhaul! This was not just a facelift; it was the equivalent of a lifeline, a desperately needed boost.

In a few weeks our space was looking sharp, inviting and cozy and it boosted morale. There was something about Keith, he had a heart for families, he was passionate, generous and his son Kevin was no different. They embraced our organization and gradually became part of our extended family. It was a ray of hope that would turn out to be complete sunshine! They stopped in from time to time to chat with me, and with the team, and they helped relieve some of my stress. I was also able to share with them my vision of moving premises and they embraced it, also agreeing to help.

Now that our centre was looking lovely, we added a "Welcome" sign in bright colours with animals hidden between the letters. The children that came to the centre loved it. They loved the zebra, the lion and the toucan the most. The reception area was bright, it felt welcoming and the atmosphere was much lighter than it had been. We had caught a break, but just as we were getting into the swing of the new look, along came another contraction.

Mellissa, another very seasoned staff member who had been with the organization for over six years, and who had also become a trusted friend, handed me her resignation. When it rains it pours! (I needed an umbrella — no, there was too much rain for an umbrella. It's a good job I saw Arks everywhere because I needed one.) I began to wonder if they were all going to leave.

She was about to become a grandmother and she wanted to be there for her daughter. Who could begrudge her that? Once again, we suffered another loss. How much more loss could we handle? It hurt. Although I was excited for her beginning the new chapter in her life, this contraction was still painful and threatened the well-being of our baby. I asked that she stay in touch as I valued her wisdom. It seemed all too familiar. Déjà vu! We were bleeding again. At this rate I worried if we would carry this baby to term? Morale was waning despite the small wins. No one said it would be easy. The only way I knew how to handle things was to continue to persevere. I refused to give up. I hired a person to fill Mellissa's role. Rosa was the most unlikely candidate of the many I interviewed but I hired her and she ended up being an incredible asset. She was a very interesting person and brought a lot to the table. Her drive, ambition and big picture thinking would prove invaluable.

I spent more time with the team so that together we could talk, dream, and plan on the same page. It took a while for us to gel, but we did. I felt that this was definitely the team with the drive and guts to get us to the new space. Our rocky beginning gave way to a smooth half of the second trimester and our vision as a team became one. We were mid-second trimester and we felt safe enough to announce our pregnancy. We began telling our friends, our families, our community, we were going to be moving. Our due date was summer of the next year, at least at that was the plan.

Perception

Your reality is as you perceive it to be. So, it is true, that by altering this perception, we can alter our reality.

– William Constantine

Our round belly was showing we had announced to the whole world that we would be moving. I am glad that no one asked us where, because I didn't know where yet, there were a few other things to take care of before then.

One of the first things I wanted to change about Anna's House was its name and people's perception of it. Every time I mentioned my new job and where I worked to anyone in the community, no one seemed to know anything about the organization, despite the fact that it had existed for twelve years. It was hidden and tucked away in the community. Our name did not say who we were or what we did. Our organization was started in 2000 and was named after Dr. Anna Schilstra, Steinbach's first female physician, who specialized in obstetrics in the early

1900s. Initially the organization looked after only young low-income families and children. As our services expanded there was no advertising to communicate to our community how the range of services and participants had changed as such our name became synonymous with single moms on welfare, poverty-stricken, marginalized and low-income families. Other families that needed our help felt they could not come to us because they were not all on low incomes. Women with serious issues such as postpartum depression, for whom we offered classes, did not feel they could attend the centre, this was very concerning.

Your name is your brand; it's part of your social DNA. Your name identifies who you are and where you belong and often begins to tell your story before you do. Disney conjures up a certain image in your mind as does Cadbury, Shell Oil, Sheraton Hotels, Honda, Jeep, Apple, Black & Decker and Heinz to name a few. Their names stand for who they are and what they do. People's perception of them is their reality. It may not be the truth but it is their truth and our community's perception of us was simply not true. Whether we like it or not, people will always judge a book by its cover. In business an organization will first be judged by its name and logo, which are the external representations of the organization. The same was true for us. Our name was Anna's House and our logo was a green tree. Our name did not convey who we were or what we did and neither did the logo. We could have been a tea house, greenhouse or a spa. Many people often came into the centre and asked if we were a shelter, a coffee house, a spa, or a restaurant. It was funny at first and then it became annoying because it happened on a daily basis and gave credence to the fact that no one knew what we were. The community was confused about what we did and our name did not help. Our full legal name was Anna's House Family Resource Centre Inc. For some reason the "family resource centre" part of our name got lost and as a result a very significant part of our identity got lost too.

People hear a name and a picture is created in their minds even before they see you. We all want a name that truly represents who we are, whether it's personal or professional. It took a while to choose my children's names. It took months of contemplation on the meanings of the names, how the child would be impacted and how they would be seen or perceived. It was no different for Anna's House. Much had gone into choosing its original name but now we had to change our name in order to move our organization forward and be relevant to the community we served.

There was another more pressing reason to change our name. In our local community there was a women's shelter called Agape House. Women were mistaking us for the shelter. Women facing domestic violence were coming to us by mistake. I didn't want to continue the risk of that happening, as they may be too scared to venture out again for help. I also found another new shelter that was going to be opening called Today House. With "house" in our name, it made sense for the community to think we were a shelter too. There was also the fact that another organization in town had a very similar logo (a green tree). Our logo had resulted from a high school competition run before my time. I did not want to offend anyone but the logo did not represent what we did, and it had been changed four other times in the last ten years.

Something had to be done; both logo and name should go hand in hand. There was a disconnection between our two most significant external emblems and it was apparent to the community. Unfortunately for me there was also a lot of sentimental value attached to both by the staff team and a few founding board members. But after much research and many discussions, the board agreed to a change of name and logo.

I remember several years ago I read about an experiment carried out by a group of professionals to prove the impact a name can have. A business professional told his colleagues that he had just hired a beautiful young personal assistant and he asked his colleagues if they would take her out to lunch. Her name was Harriet Pinklestein. Ninety percent of them declined. Two weeks later he asked them the same question only his new assistant was now Judy Collins, fifty-two percent of them agreed to take her out based on her name alone. Harriet and Judy were the same person. A name could attract or repel, it all has to do with perception. I took a look at some name branding and logo changes just to see how much it could cost us. I looked at organizations like Coca-Cola, Pepsi, and Exxon. I was shocked at the price range I found — up to $1.2B. Pepsi's logo change cost $1M. Did you know that the Nike swoosh cost only $35? The Twitter logo was bought off of iStock for $15 and the Google logo cost nothing — that was very encouraging, much closer to my budget of a few hundred dollars. We could change our name and logo and rebrand ourselves within our means. I patterned our name change after some of the biggest and best companies without the huge cost. The research I did helped us avoid some of the mistakes they had made.

We went about the change by asking the community first. We created a competition via the local radio station and asked the community to suggest a new name for us and the reason for their choice. We offered a really lovely prize as an incentive and the games began. It was a great opportunity to engage the community and learn more about their perception of us while getting their involvement. Names started coming in and they told us exactly what the community thought of us — a glorified daycare for moms on welfare. The competition also served as survey tool and the information we gained was invaluable. That competition was one of the best things we did. To get something you have never had you have to do something that you have never done. We heard the community loud and clear.

During the competition I spent some time looking at family resource centres in Canada and how they were named. Most of them were named after the places where they were located. So choosing the winner of the competition was easy. The winning name was "Steinbach Family Resource Centre." It had a ring to it. It spoke of our local area. Next was the logo. I hired a local printing firm to work on the logo. Designs went back and forth many times. I looked at many different options and none of them seemed right. At one point I thought the graphic artists were going to quit. I had turned down all the options presented and I was beginning to lose hope that we would ever find the right one. I had draft after draft after draft and involved my staff all the way. What they had to say was important, they were part of the process and they valued the fact that I heard their voices. We had a huge opportunity to start over and I did not want to have to do this again. Most of the big companies I had studied changed their names and logos only once unless they merged with another organization. We could not afford for this to go badly. I saw it as a chance to make history and I grabbed it with both hands. The whole process took about six to nine months — it was like having another baby!

Finally, the graphic artist presented one more option, when I saw it I knew it was the one. It showed a father, a mother and a little baby enclosed in a heart shape. Eureka! That was it. We didn't have a $1.8B budget but we did have the million-dollar logo that was going to work for us. After many months, we had our Pepsi! Now the work of rebranding could begin.

Most non-profit organizations are more concerned about the work they do than the way they look. It's understandable because when you are on the front lines it is easy to dismiss such things as branding, logos and public relations. What matters more on Monday morning at 9:00 a.m. — what to do when there is a young family in distress in your lobby, or work on a logo? I agree and I hear you but I cannot stress enough that they go hand in hand. Think about what makes you support an organization. You cannot deny that your impression of the organization plays a part. No matter how much good work you are doing, if you cannot show me how it is being done in an inviting professional way then you lose me, even though I believe in your cause. I have to have a positive perception of you and some of that starts with your face, which is your name and logo.

As soon as we made the change our perception of ourselves began to change. I sent the new logo to friends and family worldwide, everyone who saw it got it. Our new logo told our story before we did, it said what we did and how. Our message was very clear, we were all about family.

Place

A leader takes people where they want to go. A great leader takes people where they don't want to go but ought to be.

– Rosalynn Carter

We were very excited to finally have a new name and logo; it was a breath of fresh air. The logo looked very professional and the name intentional. My staff team and I had all been part of the long creative process; it was a team effort. I listened to what they had to say and it was fun to see them fully engaged. They had some of the best ideas and together we created the face of the new Steinbach Family Resource Centre. It was now time to find the right location and home for our organization. Now that I had the staff's total buy-in it made the journey a little easier. We did not have any extra funding so I delved into our existing finances in detail. We had a small amount of savings that we had asked for permission from the Canada Revenue Agency to save towards a building purchase or renovation — approximately

$50,000 saved over ten years. In Steinbach that was not enough to buy a chicken coop.

It didn't stop me from looking for properties that I thought were suitable; everything was financially out of our reach, beyond our scope but not out of our dreams. So dream I did. Dreaming was free and I did a lot of it. I made many enquires and found that there was nothing available. I refused to be discouraged, there had to be something out there. I stopped looking at what we had and what we didn't have and began to look at what we could have. I had doors slammed in my face too many times to worry about; I wondered if "NO" was my middle name. (One of my friends says "NO ah!" that's how she says the Girl Noah came about). I have always held on to the notion that the word NO is a precursor to fulfilled dreams. Every visionary has a trunk full of NO's and a slew of "crazies."

Once again I began to cast vision with my team and talked to them about more possibilities. I didn't remind them of our present state but instead I focused on where we could be. Remember Cinderella? Yes, we were dreaming of the handsome prince even though we were still dressed in rags; we needed more than a pumpkin carriage and fairy godmother — we needed a miracle, and a big one at that.

After much searching I found a property that was a little out of the main core of town. It was an old restaurant with a football field beside it, very promising. I was hopeful. They were asking $400,000. I burst out laughing at the price tag — really? We didn't have anything close to that amount. It turns out that it also used to be an old gas station and there were restrictions on the change of use. The board dismissed that opportunity and rightfully so; it was back to the drawing board. A few months later I heard of a company selling its business; the land was a prime spot for our organization. It was barely five minutes from where we were and I had dreams of perhaps adding a Starbucks to one side of the property one day, but it was too big and they wanted $800,000. The board chairperson came to see it; she liked it too but there was no way we could afford it. It was back to square one again. I was frustrated but I had to be patient and believe that the perfect property would show up soon.

Patience, they say is a virtue. I was having trouble being virtuous. All I saw and heard confirmed that property in Steinbach was expensive and that nothing was available. No one was selling a property that we could afford. I met up with a friend and shared my frustrations and she said, almost off the cuff, why don't you lease? We were currently leasing and could not afford to buy, so leasing a better space seemed to make sense. So I engaged a realtor to help me look for a property that we could lease, but there was still nothing suitable in our price range.

Between the middle of the second trimester and middle of the third trimester, you become tired and irritated easily. Doing the things that you do take a lot more effort, you get bigger, the baby gets bigger and the stretch marks are more apparent, we were in that space. One of the beautiful things about being pregnant is being able to dream about what the baby is going to look like and planning the nursery, and the further along the pregnancy the higher the anticipation.

There are days when you wish the baby would just arrive as the discomforts are increased but who wants a premature baby? So you stay the course, focus on the joy coming. We had to find a place soon.

A few weeks later one of the volunteers asked if I had seen a "for lease" sign up in town. I hadn't — it turns out that I had been driving past it every day for three months and had not seen it. She had to take me to where it was because even after she described it I couldn't see it in my mind's eye. I had not noticed the sign. The building was drab and grey... inconspicuous. It looked like an old warehouse. It had barbed wire around a yard area making it look like a mini-prison that fell out of the 1970s. Can someone say ugly? Seriously, ugly is kind!

I contacted my realtor and went to see it the same day. When I got inside it was love at first sight (I could hear violins), I can't tell you why. I literally fell in love with the building. It truly was downright ugly but somehow I could see its potential; I had a niggly that this was it. The "décor" was from the 1970s, a mustardy colour throughout. There was some ceramic tile in the front entrance, a small glass cage and a reception that hogged too much space. It was divided into a million small offices and the carpets were moggy and it was dark and dingy with very few windows. It was really nasty to say the least. A company that sold animal feed had just left. One third of the building was a garage with ten-foot garage doors. Most people would have turned away, but I could see what a great building it could be. I had to try very hard to contain my excitement. I could barely breathe. I had finally found the space that we needed to be in. I had a vision of what it could be. I could see it two years down the road in my mind's eye. It looked great!

My realtor probably thought I was crazy, what was new? We did some preliminary calculations and with some additional donations and financial planning, we could afford it. However, we would have to overhaul the building and I had no idea how. Finding the space was step number one and we had to take it one step at a time. I remember being worried when I was first pregnant with Miqaela; I wondered how we were ever going to afford a child. With help and support from friends and family it worked itself out somehow. With the board, donors and community support and the necessary due diligence, this would be no different. I skipped back to the office to tell my staff team. They were curious about their team leader's singing and the new spring in my step.

I excitedly called the board and asked if they would come and see it. I was beyond happy. I found it! It was pretty close to the feeling I had when that pregnancy stick turned pink... positive... What I always knew was possible suddenly seemed within reach. No one would believe that a tiny organization like ours could even think about being in a bigger facility. Well here we were on the threshold of change and I was excited. I could barely sit!

I brought in a building contractor to estimate how much money it would cost to renovate the building. We thought of doing a partial renovation and keeping some of the existing offices... it would not be great but certainly manageable. It was going to be in the region of $75,000. We had $50,000 so we would have to raise $25,000. That didn't seem too bad. I felt that if we were going to all this trouble anyway then why not renovate the whole building? (I know… my Noah head!) I brought in another set of professional building contractors and they estimated the entire renovation would be in excess of $350,000 — that was an insane amount of money. I wouldn't let my mind believe that it was impossible.

I will never forget hearing about an interview with Carl Lewis, the great American former track and field athlete. He was asked, when preparing for his next high jump competition whether he thought what he was attempting was impossible. He said he never let his mind go there because such thinking had a way of getting to his feet. Me too, such thinking would have a way of getting to my heart.

A few days later our monthly board meeting came up and the board decided to meet at the property. I was like the proverbial kid in the candy store. I showed them around excitedly and waited with bated breath for the response. Individually they each took a good look around. It was very obvious that I was passionate and proud, akin to making a pregnancy announcement. I waited for their reply. It came, but it was not what I was expecting. I was truly shocked when they all categorically told me NO! They had a million reasons why it was not practical and on top of all that we did not have much money and could not afford it! My heart sank. They had a negative response for every idea, possibility or opportunity I raised. They were dead set against it. I went home that night dejected, torn and just stuck. I knew in my heart that we had to move or I would have to. That made me really sad; I loved the work we were doing but I knew it would only be a matter of time before I left the organization because there was no way forward. I had a twenty-five-minute drive home. Usually my vehicle is pumping with loud music. (Yes, I am one of those!) That evening it was a quiet drive home. I needed to plan the next move. I felt so many emotions, from sadness to anger. I was upset; this was the third building that had been rejected. I have to say that the previous two rejections were valid but this one wasn't, at least I didn't think so. How do you tell your boss that this was a deal breaker without making it sound like a threat? I got home and took many deep breaths. All I can tell you is that my minivan holds many a secret. I express my thoughts aloud in my vehicle. If my steering wheel could speak I would be in big trouble. (Don't think of me like that — I am sure your car holds some secrets too!)

Something in me would not give. I knew it would only be a matter of time before the property would be swooped up. So I did what I always do. I prayed and got some advice. I needed a miracle! Not just one board member was against the idea — all of them were, all six. Despite the battle in my mind, I had to go into work the next day pumped. I had spent the last year working really hard to get my staff to believe. They told me every director before me had promised them that they would move and here I was again about to dash their hopes. I couldn't do it. I knew I had to smile when I went into work the next day. I had buried that "plastic smile" in my bag; I put it on and cried beneath. My team asked me how the meeting went and I told them all was well. It was like the way you feel when you have to smile and welcome your spouse home from work knowing that you are going to tell him during supper that you had just had a miscarriage. I was smiling but completely miserable.

I don't know how to give up; it is not in my DNA, how could I give up now? I had come too far, I encouraged myself — who else was going to?

I called Mellissa, my former staff member and took her and a few friends to the building to show them what I was thinking, they saw it completely. There are times when you need to bring in people to keep your mind focused. They fuel your fire and keep you crazy. I would do whatever it took and if it meant losing my job in the process it was worth the cost. I would rather lose trying than live with what could have been. It wasn't about me. It was bigger than me. It was about the thousands of families that we could help now and in the future.

I could understand the board's reasoning and they had valid reasons. I knew that we did not have the money; I just needed permission to try. Every business or life venture comes to a crossroads and it takes courage to defy the odds, take risks and hope for the impossible.

I needed an ally so I went to the board chair and bared my soul. She was an amazing boss but she was in a very difficult position. She had an organization to protect. I had only been there just over a year and I was asking her to take a big risk. I am glad I was not in her shoes. I gently reminded her that they had hired me for change. This was it. Faith is spelled R.I.S.K. If we didn't take the risk nothing was going to happen. I put my job on the line. That was the only collateral I had. I knew that if this risk did not pay off I was out anyway. It was worth that much to me. Something I said must have struck a chord, she heard me. I was able to convince her to change her mind and she gave me her vote. Phew! That was close. What she didn't know was that I had two speeches prepared. If her answer to taking a risk was negative, integrity demanded that I resign. I could not function in a pair of handcuffs. Then she told me she would speak to the other board members and hopefully they would agree too. So one after the other the votes came in to go ahead. It was not unanimous but I had a majority and ran with it. I was also scared; it was a risk for me too, I had to feel the fear and do it anyway.

Around that time two very significant things happened. First we received two huge donations that helped keep hope alive. The next significant thing I didn't see coming. I got a phone call from Keith one of the guys that helped paint the old building. He said he wanted me to meet a friend of his. He gave me her phone number and the name of the company where she worked, but when I Googled it nothing came up. I didn't realize it but I had misheard the company name, so I could not do any research on who she was before I met her. I called her assistant and set up the meeting.

Chantelle was a nice lady. We chatted about this and that and learned we had a lot in common. She had just recently lost her husband and I had just lost my brother-in-law at the same time and we both had compassion for those who were less fortunate. Then she asked me the million-dollar question. "What do you want from me?" My reflex response was, "Nothing." I was happy to make a new acquaintance. I didn't know she was the CEO of a multi-million dollar building company. She seemed very shocked when I told her all that we did. I explained how amazing it was and how much of a difference we made to others. I apologized for not bringing a gift, something I usually do when I go to meetings. I told her point-blank that I wanted her heart more than a cheque as money was finite. She had to leave hurriedly to attend another meeting. I picked up the tab, left the restaurant and forgot all about it. I had tons of these meetings; I talked to anyone who had ears about what we were doing.

I went back to the office and it was business as usual until I got a call from the painters, Keith & Kevin. They asked how my meeting went with the CEO. I explained that it had gone well and that I thought she was a great lady. As things turned out she was touched by our work and had decided that her company would support us. I was thrilled. They made a sizeable donation that year around the same time I was trying to convince the board about the new property and that became a tipping point.

Time was running out on the leasing opportunity. The landlord had informed me that there were other parties interested in the property and I had to make my position permanent or walk away from the table. I called the board chair. We had to do what we had to do. I wrote a letter of intent to the property owner and things began. Having done all the negotiations, calculations, and projections we were ready to take the biggest risk ever. My heart was pounding...

It brought back vivid memories of arriving at the hospital ready to have my son. I was nervous, hands sweating, standing on the curb of the unknown. The surgeon made the cut. It was done. There was no going back. I had Michael in fifteen minutes.

My boss and I signed the lease...OMG! The deed was done and the adrenalin started pumping. There was no going back. We were now legally bound to take possession within a few months. We had passed the point of no return. I immediately changed my screensaver to the address of our new space. I saw the dream every day as I spent some of every working day visualizing where we were going to be. Our dream was coming true; we actually had a new space; now the real test would be in raising the funds for the renovations and asking the community for help. It had been almost twenty months in real time and there was still a distance to go. The ultrasounds were looking good, now we had to get to full term and then push.

Persuade

Fight for the things that you care about, but do it in a way that will lead others to join you.

- Ruth Bader Ginsberg

We were all still high from obtaining the new premises, and the reality of all the work that had to be done had not fully dawned on us. The joy of getting to the third trimester was enough. Not too long after that on an ordinary day at the office, my childcare worker called in sick and we desperately needed someone that morning to take her place. I jumped in to help. I have always run a very flat organization. We all do what needs to be done regardless of our position. My regular day of e-mails and phone calls turned into a morning of Lego bricks, toy trains and little dolls. A little girl (whom I will call Amber to protect her identity and privacy) had come in to spend time in our playroom that morning. I got down on all fours and began to play with this cute but frail little girl. She had mousy brown hair and I noticed she had thin little arms. She giggled with me but there was something sad in her eyes. Her clothes were not new — very thrift store looking — but she had a pretty face and captivating smile. I knew I had not seen her before but she seemed familiar and I really enjoyed playing with her. We giggled and laughed and had lots of fun. I specifically remember how much she loved the little Fisher Price mat we had. It was made up of a small racing track that went around a little town. Building silly things with the Lego bricks got lots of laughter from her too. I cannot explain it but we made a connection and for those sixty minutes we were in a world of our own. My director hat was gone and out came my kid hat. We played, just two kids, one big one and one very small one. It was obvious that Amber was having a lot of fun, and I was too. It is funny how a child has the unique ability to help you travel back to your own childhood. Thankfully I had not forgotten how to play. (I am convinced, as adults we should all learn to play more.) When it was time to leave she gave me the biggest hug ever. She wrapped her little arms around my neck, tears welling in her eyes. She didn't want to leave; I put it down to her enjoying herself so much. My heart ached as she cried. I cannot explain how our bond happened — it just happened and it happened quickly. Her social worker came to pick her up and she was gone. I came across dozens of children each week, why the bond with this little one? I was not sure, but I had one of those nigglies.

Amber was back the next week and I had some time to play and chat with her and her mom. Amber was usually dropped off by a social worker and her mom met her at the centre, as she did not have custodial rights. She was able to exercise her visitation rights at our centre. There was a story there but I made no judgments. Sometimes families choose to share their current parenting situation and sometimes not. We offered an environment where families could feel safe regardless. Over the next few weeks, my staff spent much more time with Amber and her mom and they began to notice some bruising on her. We initially put it down to childhood rambunctiousness. Cuts and nicks are a normal part of growing up, but then she came in next week with a black eye, the week after that it was two black eyes, we became suspicious. The following week it was bruising on the side of her face. My staff brought it to my attention once more and this time I asked to speak to her mom. Her mom explained that she was concerned for her daughter's welfare and had expressed this to the authorities. The authorities had placed the child in a foster home for a reason and I was not privy to that information, and legally I could not pry, but it seemed obvious that she was still not safe. I was getting worried, this whole situation was very concerning, but my primary concern was to give Amber a voice.

Incidentally, the newspaper headlines that week made this matter more concerning. The papers reported that after a lengthy investigation, the recommendations on the Phoenix Sinclair case were now public. Phoenix Victoria Hope Sinclair was a young child that had been neglected, abused and eventually murdered by her mother and stepfather while in contact with social services. Everyone was on edge. She was only five — too young to have lost her life in this way. I was not sure what to do about Amber. I had no idea where her bruises came from; her mom felt she was being abused in the foster home. It was a very messy situation and my lawyer head was looking for answers — I could not help but get involved.

The straw that broke the camel's back occurred a few weeks later. Amber came in to play as usual and she had bruising that looked as if someone had grabbed her by the face — bluish-black imprints of five fingers. It looked really bad. So I asked her what happened to her face and in her little gentle voice she said her foster parents hurt her, that is all I had to hear. I was truly upset. I had seen enough. It was my legal obligation to report to the authorities when a child's safety was in jeopardy. I had sworn an oath when receiving my citizenship that I would uphold the laws of this great nation, one of them being to report to the authorities if I suspected a child was in danger. I took my oath seriously plus I had to be able to look at myself in the mirror every day. I had personally observed the increased injury to this child. I talked to the worker that brought her in, her response shocked me, she had no idea how Amber had got the bruising. To make matters worse, alarm bells went off when we had given Amber a serving of fishy crackers and milk as we do for all participants, which she gladly ate. But she was still hungry, even after she ate more than three servings. She was too small to be eating so much; it was obvious she was extremely hungry; something was not right. What hurt the most was that she was too fragile and small to be experiencing so much pain. She couldn't possibly weigh more than twenty pounds and she was almost four years old.

I was going to get to the bottom of this matter so I started making some phone calls. (I have had to leave out some significant details of the case for privacy reasons. My goal in telling this story is not to point fingers or castigate anyone.

Somewhere along the line the authorities failed, but so did the community, and if I didn't do anything then that would include me. I couldn't live with that. There is an African proverb that says "When two elephants fight it's the grass that suffers." In my business often that grass is a child. My fight was to prevent the fight; the casualties were too costly.) I made more phone calls, but I felt I was being stonewalled; there was a lot of red tape. I didn't get it. I felt like no one was listening. There was a brick wall at every turn, I followed procedure and still nothing. I tried the polite way but I was not getting anywhere. It was time for crazy! I had to get someone's attention.

I recalled the case of Victoria Adjo Climbie, an eight-year-old Ivorian girl who was tortured and murdered by her guardians in the United Kingdom back in 2000. It was a huge case. One hundred and six professionals were in touch with her and her guardians and none of them saw the danger she was in until she died. She ultimately died of hypothermia in a house that had central heating. A huge investigation followed that highlighted all the systemic failures, but it was too late for Victoria. All it would have taken is for one professional to have cared enough and the results could be have been different.

It was not too late for Amber. So crazy began with me sending the Victoria Climbie video to the authorities with a note about Amber saying I refuse to be one of the one hundred and six who did nothing. I was ready for war and they had no idea what I was ready and willing to do to save a child's life. They must have thought me insane, and they were right. (I am sure my name is a swear word for some of the authorities to this day, and frankly speaking, I don't care.) I wanted the authorities to take note. I will say that along this journey I came across two very special social workers that were extremely helpful. They know who they are.

I never really knew how deeply hurt about this I was until one night I woke up in the middle of the night and my husband asked me what was wrong. I explained that I could not sleep because my heart hurt. I had two children who were tucked away safe in their beds and I had one child who was out there and in trouble. The only difference between my two children and Amber was a birth canal. There is an African proverb that says a child who is the same age as your own child is also your child. A life was at stake and like every mama bear whose cubs are being threatened my claws were out. After having called the authorities and getting no real response, I called the Child Advocate office to air my concern and explain the situation. The last time I saw Amber she was frail and bruised. Particularly shocking were the little marks on her right wrist. She was pinching herself. I was told much later that this was how she coped. She would pinch herself to deal with hunger pangs or any other pain.

I saw Amber later that day. When it was time to leave she came to hug me and began to really cry, lots of tears falling down her little face. She begged me to keep her and I felt powerless. I hugged her frail body feeling all the emotions a mom feels who is losing her child, and it was painful. I whispered into her little ears, "I promise I will get you out, I don't know how but I promise to get you out." I said, "I love you!" She refused to let me go. Her little bony arms hugged my neck tighter. I literally had to peel her hands off of me. She was screaming at this point. "I love you Vicki," she kept saying, and those were her last words as her worker pulled her off me; it broke my heart. Here I was, this strong tough executive director yet I was powerless. I hate being powerless. "My child" was being taken away and I couldn't stand it. I could hear the numbers counting down all over again 10...9... I was ready to fight for this child. The new round one had already begun.

The authorities and those around me made the mistake of thinking that I was her mom's friend. But this was very personal; Amber was my personal friend and she had a powerful friend in me. Winning against infertility gives you the right qualifications to fight.

Every day I pushed and made phone calls and talked to anyone who had ears. I persuaded all who heard me. It became our mission to rescue this little one and rescue her we did.

During all this time, Amber had made me a Froot Loop necklace and drawn me a picture, which was on my wall. Call me crazy but I read the picture. It had all kinds of colour stickers but it also had some happy faces. Every one of those faces was upside down except for one. It felt like she was trying to tell me something and I was listening. I could not shake off my feelings. I called the Child Advocate again. I made it very clear that I was sure she would die in a few days if help did not come soon. Thankfully, I got hold of someone who really heard me and things were put in motion to investigate the situation immediately. I was able to present a very strong case and the Child Advocate ordered a medical exam. They did a full and thorough examination of all her bruises and were horrified at the results. She was removed from the foster home immediately. For a while I did not know where she was, the authorities could not tell me that. Then I got the call and learned that she was being placed in a new foster home. It was bittersweet news because it meant I would not see her again as her new home was far away, but the most important thing was that she was safe. It had taken a while to get her out but I had fulfilled my promise to my friend. I cried. We had won! As the phone call ended it suddenly dawned on me why she looked so familiar, Amber's story personified our centre's story; we were small and not very significant, we didn't have much economically but we had heart, we just needed to be heard. She was our story of hope and it demonstrated the power of a team and what we could accomplish by working together. It also displayed what our centre could do for the community if given the chance.

Everywhere I went I told our story very passionately and persuasively and people began to listen. They began to make donations to help all the other little Ambers we would come into contact with. Our new space would make that possible on a greater scale, they also began to understand what we were about. We had caught the community's attention. We not only had a persuasive story, we had one that was powerful, compelling and with a happy ending. We were persuaded, now we could persuade others. The results would speak for themselves.

Power

Culture can become a 'secret weapon' that makes extraordinary things happen.

– Jon Katzenbach

We now had some support from local builders and small pockets of the community but there were still other areas of the community that we needed to reach. We needed to help ourselves and tell our community about what we were doing. Stephen Covey's principle in *Seven Habits of Highly Effective People* helped me analyze the situation best: "Understand before you can be understood." I took a step back and tried to look at our organization from both inside out and outside in and I discovered that internally we needed to shift the way we thought about who we were. A close look revealed that a "poverty mentality" had bled into our culture. We accepted willingly that we were poor and as an organization not good enough to have anything nice (except the Clothing Café). The way we spoke, the way we dealt with the public betrayed how we felt about ourselves. There was nothing wrong with helping some low-income families, or those on welfare — it was the way we did that did not provide dignity to our participants, we were apologetic about what we did. There was power in what we did but we didn't see it that way.

I believe that every organization or individual can be powerful, in fact very powerful if they can find a way to tap into it.

I looked at the many things we did in the community that no one else did. We guided families having babies and we helped them look after their children from the ages zero to five, which is a very vulnerable time for any family. [According to our regional health authority there were over twelve hundred babies born in the area annually.] We had the unique opportunity to spend time with at least one third of those babies each year. We were the only family resource centre in all of South Eastman, which meant we covered over twenty different localities. We offered a variety of classes for new mothers and young children, pregnant teens, and parents; we were the leading community organization for classes in understanding post-partum depression. No other organization did this. I recognized what made us unique; that was power, and now we had to capitalize on it, package it, present it, use it and own it.

The easiest way to do this was to examine our own culture and as they say take our own inventory. We had to do an ultrasound and take an in-depth look at ourselves. An ultrasound was the best way to see what was happening on the inside. I was always fascinated that it was possible to see the baby, find out its gender and monitor growth. Sometimes it revealed problems that could be dealt with in utero.

My ultrasound examination revealed that our mindset produced our culture and that translated into everything we did. We offered help to others but we needed help to see how amazing we were and the difference we were making. I could not accept or work with a culture centered on poverty-thinking, settling for always being in need. It was in direct contradiction to the person I am. It was time for change. If we could change our culture it would seep into everything we did and ultimately change the whole organization.

I asked a lot of questions. I learned that the staff team was uncomfortable with media or asking for help from the community. Our culture was an assault on growth or progress of any kind. So I got to work the next day and asked my team if we as an organization had ever given anything to any of the businesses in town. There was the look of surprise, the "we are the ones in need why would we give anything away" look. The answer was an emphatic "NO." It made my point. They say to get something you have never had you have to do something you have never done. We were about to do something we had never done. I had an idea — a crazy concept.

In a bid to radically change things I announced to the team that we were going to give back to our community and thank them for all they had done so far and tell them about all the wonderful things that we did. It was time to remind them that we were unique and we made lives better in our community. Can you imagine the response? They thought it was a crazy idea. We were not rich in resources but we were all very resourceful and many of our gifts and talents were untapped. I began to look at the things that were working, what did we do well? One thing that we did really well was bake. In order to keep our costs down we made most of the snacks we served from scratch. We baked cookies, cheese biscuits, scones, and other delicious goodies. Our building was always filled with the aroma of fresh, sumptuous, delicious baking.

Every one of us has something to give and every organization has something it can give. I used to believe that only big companies with huge reserves were able to give to others. It is simply not true. It is easy to think about your size and equate it to your ability to help others, but that would be erroneous thinking. Being "poor" is no crime, it is a state of being, but a poverty mentality is a state of mind which is much more dangerous and I believe it was holding our organization hostage from moving to the next level. I announced that we were going to bake four thousand cookies and give them away to the local businesses that had given us donations or had been involved with us in the past. My staff team was not happy. It was a lot more work than they wanted to take on. I could see this as the beginning of great things and a shift in our culture but I didn't have their buy-in. Even though my staff didn't agree with me they had seen what they now called "my crazy" produce results, so they very reluctantly got on board. They were not very enthusiastic. I thought my bookkeeper was going to have a conniption when she learned that it would cost $300 – $400 to do this. I could "hear" her thoughts, "we don't have enough money and now you want to give money away." I tried to explain that it was the only way I knew how to get money, plus it was important for us to show appreciation for all that we had already received, it was great for public relations too. She didn't believe me. There was really no more economical way to stand out and say thank you. Most organizations gave cards, we did too but our home-baked treats came from our hearts and hands to the community.

As life would have it a few days later, I was called to our reception desk and there was Michelle. After a brief discussion it came to light that she had been depressed for over five years and had finally found better ways to cope. She wanted to volunteer her time and as usual I asked her what she was good at. Her response was music to my ears, she said baking. Yay! She was the quintessential baker, so much so that she even had her KitchenAid mixer in the trunk of her car. Michelle was nothing short of amazing. She was a very analytical baker; everything was measured and precise. Long story short, she baked 4000 cookies, and each one was the same size and weight! It was pure "cookieville" for a long time at the centre. My staff team was still unsure; no one said it was going to be easy.

My motive in all this was to begin a culture of saying "thank you" for everything. I believe that as a non-profit organization/ registered charity you cannot keep asking and taking. It was on that premise that our culture of appreciation was born. It wasn't just with cookies, we began to say thank you by e-mail, snail mail, social media, radio, and the local newspaper for everything we received. As Michelle baked we packaged the cookies. (Packaging has been a passion of mine since I was a kid, I could make a one-dollar cookie packet look like a million bucks.) My staff was not happy at the prospect of dealing with all the cookies even if I now had someone to bake them — 4000 of them. We bought simple low-cost white boxes and the plastic inserts for food as required by the CIFA. We had scrapbooking supplies that had been donated and a whole lot of bling and ribbon from the dollar store. We decorated the boxes whenever we could. While on the phone to save time, we were sticking stones and butterflies on boxes and we made huge bows. The boxes looked so shi-shi-foo-foo that even the company we bought the white boxes from put one of them on display. We had given them some cookies too. They could not believe what we turned a thirty-five-cent box into. Presentation is everything. We made a small box of cookies look amazing; some of our power was in making something so little look so great — and it felt great!

I became the "Cookie Girl" in town, delivering cookies to our sponsors and donors. Most companies were happy; there were a few that were leery, but all in all people were happy to receive them. Many offices enjoyed the cookies and fought over the boxes, some had to raffle off the boxes because their staff members wanted them. In some offices, I got a cautious "what do you want" look; others didn't treat me well. I had our families on my mind so it didn't matter. We just wanted to say thank you! And we did. Since then we have given away candy, cupcakes and cards and now we always say thank you!

It didn't seem logical for a non-profit organization to give back because most of us essentially beg for money, but I did not want to be one of those; we were here to make a difference on every level. I still had to watch the costs; I didn't want donors to think we were wasting their money, because we weren't. I just wanted to change our culture, the way our non-profit organization operated, and more importantly how our community viewed us. It took a while to catch on and we used every free method we could find to show our appreciation, and sometimes a little cookie dough. We have found very simple inexpensive ways to say "Thank you" and continue to do so to this day. We appealed to companies and businesses for donations of merchandise that we could use as appreciation gifts, it was a win-win.

Our decision to say thank you slowly began to change people's perception of us; it changed our culture and ultimately changed our organization. "Thank you" — two words I believe literally changed our world. I knew it was right but I didn't understand the impact of it until I began to tell our story in the community. We became a powerful organization by being able to say thank you, tell our story and explain the services and programs that we provide. We tapped into what we already had and became a little powerhouse.

Consequently, we engaged the community and the donations for the new facility began to come in, and in larger amounts than we could ever have imagined.

Plan

Ordinary people believe only in the possible. Extraordinary people visualize not what is possible or probable but rather what is impossible. And by visualizing the impossible they begin to see it as possible.

– Charles Carter Scott

Christmas came and went and that winter was long and brutally cold! December and January were tough months. I remember it was extremely cold. The temperature sat at -40°C and lower most days, and with the wind chill it was almost unbearable. There was not a building contractor in sight; they could not work outside because everything was frozen solid. My fundraising efforts were just as cold. Before I knew it, February had arrived and the first rent cheque was due... and work on the renovation had not begun. The board chair was nervous signing that rent cheque, especially when not one brick or tile had been moved yet. We were essentially paying rent in two places. I talked to potential donors at every opportunity and I was at the building every day. I wrote newspaper articles to create awareness about the project. I walked around and dreamed and hosted tours for prospective donors to get their perspective on the space and also to keep the dream alive.

It was time for us to get to work on the new building plans, I engaged an architectural firm to discuss our needs and the possibilities. It was clear that it was going to be quite the process; there were so many things to consider. It's a good thing that most of the times you have a big dream you have more optimism and enthusiasm than sense. The enormity of the project did not dawn on me until we actually began planning. I got to know every nook and cranny of our new space and I took our wish list with all the things we dreamed for our new space. It was the list on our wall that I had asked our staff team to fill up with their dreams and wishes if money were no object. I took the list with me to the meetings with the architects; I didn't want to forget anything. I spent a good week consulting with the firm explaining our vision. They came back with a great design concept, it was very "shi-shi-foo-foo" — beautiful from a designer's perspective but it would cost a fortune to pull off. It had all the things we wanted but it blew our tentative renovation budget right out the window! The architects' plans were very upmarket and based on their calculations it was going to cost in excess of $600,000. That was completely out of the question so we had to change the plan to a more basic design that was more affordable. No rounded corners or high-tech millwork. Every decision had cost effectiveness at its core. With the help of local draftsmen I modified the plan, but even with the modified plan the price tag was in the $300,000 range.

I took the modified drawings and used them as a tool for casting vision and fundraising. It was slow going until Chantelle, the CEO that I had previously met for coffee, called me out of the blue. She said she had been thinking of a way to help; she had an idea and she introduced me to her design team. Her company was a very successful building firm with heart and a commitment to improving the community. She had me close to tears when she told me her idea; she decided to hold a breakfast on our behalf. She would invite all her affiliates, tradesmen, designers, and engineers out for breakfast. She asked that I just share our centre's story. I was floored.

It was set for a few weeks later — 7:00 a.m. at a local restaurant. I made special arrangements with my kids' daycare to drop them off at 6:45 a.m. I put the pedal to the metal and got there as soon as I could. I arrived at 7:15am. It was very simple, we all got some food and when it was time to speak I had fifteen minutes to tell our story. I told Amber's story along with our own and the need for a safe place for all the moms and kids in our area. I didn't have a speech written I just spoke from my heart. Twenty-five contractors had come. I finished speaking and sat down, I was too nervous to eat my muffin. Afterwards every one of those men came up to me and said, "I'm in." They were going to help in one way or another. Chantelle's company would donate the project management. I was overwhelmed, help had come and things were actually going to be OK. It still meant having to do some fundraising, but with this kind of support already in place, I knew we could do it.

At that time, I brought the whole staff team to the new space. I explained all the wonderful things that were going to happen from the mental pictures I had painted. I was very excited for them to see the dream coming together. They came into the building and I waited for the excited screams of joy. They never came. Instead some of them were bickering over where their offices were going to be, the awful colour and where the light switches were situated. I was stunned. I thought if anyone would get this, my staff team would. It reminded me of some of the comments people made when I was going through infertility; I knew they meant well and had good intentions but some things they said were very insensitive and extremely hurtful. They say, "It's lonely at the top." It sure was. I am sure every visionary goes through this. I was out there in the freezing cold, fundraising and raising awareness and some of the team I was doing it for didn't understand it. It was a hard pill to swallow. (Looking back I realize that it was difficult for them to "see" what I saw and I now understand their initial scepticism.) As sad as I was about it, it helped me strategize how to move forward. I chose to spend a lot more of my time discussing the building with people who were dreamers like me. I literally put an imaginary red circle around negative minds. Negative talk had a way of literally getting to your feet in sub-zero temperatures.

Around that time, I had the good fortune to meet Judy Peters, a local reporter. Unknown to me, she had been a previous participant at Anna's House several years before. She knew the old premises and when she saw the new building, she loved it even in its ugly state. She could see the possibilities too. Every opportunity she got to tell our story in the local paper she did.

Renovations began in March when the weather became warmer and as with all renovations, we found things we did not expect. The building was in worse shape than we originally thought. The thoughts of doing a partial renovation died quickly. We had to gut it. It was grungy and the carpets were threadbare. It was divided into too many small cubicle-type offices. Thankfully I worked with the most amazing site and project managers. Big Don was on site daily. We talked in detail about every door, window and wall. Don was physically huge, he was about seven feet tall, but was the nicest giant that I had ever met and we worked very well together. He was very respectful considering I knew nothing about building. I had built a house but this was a behemoth in comparison. As for the project manager, Mitch, I might as well have called him Dad. He treated me like his daughter. I learned more about building from these two amazing leaders than I ever had before. Together we came up with a plan to implement the simplified drawings and list of suppliers. We cut back on luxuries and went for durable, functional and cost-effective. We brought people to the site and toured them to show what we had done and to see if they could help. There was a buzz of activity every day. Both Mitch and Don introduced me to many vendors and other professionals. Working with them so closely, I gathered so much information, they left no stone unturned in my education. The most important thing was sticking to the plans we had.

We all had specific roles to play. They kept me on track while being very patient with me. I had to remove my director hat and become a building project manager apprentice. They could see that I was hungry to learn and at the same time I was willing to do anything to help finish the centre. I asked and answered a million questions or so it seemed. Every time a technician, inspector, tradesman or labourer came to the site it was an opportunity to share our story and our plans and I never missed an opportunity. Unless they had had personal contact with the centre before, all the tradesmen and visitors to the work site were fascinated by our story. I recall someone who worked in insurance came by and after I shared our story with him, not only did he have his company help us with a sizeable donation he made a personal commitment and gave us four new doors for the building. Don, Mitch and I coordinated most of the in-kind giving which consisted of lumber, paint, drywall, and other building supplies. I took about a thousand pictures so I could capture all the wonderful memories and moments of the build. In the middle of it all I had media come in and make a walk-through video so the community could watch it on YouTube. I am pleased to say that things went according to plan and there were no injuries on the project. I continued to celebrate the daily changes from moving the entrance to cutting new windows to creating a new reception. The building was transforming and looking more like the drawings with each passing day.

The tradesmen who had attended the breakfast came out at different times. Most of them gave in-kind by way of their labour or materials. This made a huge impact on the project. What I was attempting to do was crazy, a $300,000 renovation with $50,000 in the bank. I planned the best way I knew how and then I let our community know about it. Our fundraising efforts moved from $25,000 to $300,000. I talked about our plans to anyone who would listen. I had a plan, drawings and passion. It was possible, it could be done. I could not settle for anything less than that. I had once heard a quote by Don Ward: "If the dream is big enough the facts don't count." I was about to prove it.

Patience

No matter how great the talents or efforts, some things take time. You cannot produce a baby in one month by getting nine women pregnant.

– Warren Buffet

I was in the new building every day. I was there to drop off coffee for the men working on the project, check the progress and take a ton of pictures. It was a very exciting time! I am sure that my car could drive to the new building all by itself. I worked in two places — both the old building and the new. It was nothing to drive to the new building ten times in one day. I had to be there at a moment's notice if the building contractors had a question. I worked hand in hand with the project manager and as the work progressed I asked for donations of building supplies on behalf of our children. People have often asked me why I was so bold. It was easy; every parent would do the same. I had the children who used our centre on my mind. You might be embarrassed asking for money and supplies for yourself but when it comes to your child you will do anything. They say the difference between a mommy and a bulldog is lipstick. I maintain that I have both the lipstick and the tenacity of a bulldog.

The third trimester is the most tiring part of a pregnancy; it is the time when everyone knows you are pregnant because your belly is so big it is hard to hide. We were not hiding. We wanted the whole world to know. We were glowing and anticipating a safe birth. We could faintly see the finish line ahead. In a few months' it would be time to push.

I asked for lumber, eaves troughs, bricks, tin, toilets, sinks, you name it. I asked for what we needed and I enjoyed every minute of it. Did I get a few more gray hairs? Absolutely. Stress levels were high but I persevered. There were no guarantees that the donations were going to come in, but they came in at a steady pace, though not as fast as I would have liked. Although I had the support of the board and the staff team, there were many times when I felt alone on the frontlines because it was a constant uphill climb. I just kept putting one foot in front of the other and when I couldn't walk, I crawled, but I kept moving, believing that it was going to happen. I had to be patient.

I fondly remember a few moments along the way. Watching during the two days it took to frame the building was so cool — very similar to that first baby kick — and I could finally see what the drawings looked like in real life. I walked into my office in its skeletal form with just the studs up and it already felt like home. Seeing the changes every day was breathtaking. What would seem like ordinary changes to most people were incredible to me.

Some of those moments were fun things we did, which also added to our collection of gratitude moments and excited memories. The first day the lights were connected, we compared it to the moment in New York City when the Christmas tree lights are switched on. Especially memorable was the day we pressed the disabled access button and the door opened — preceded by our hand drum rolls. Providing wheelchair access to families was one of my proudest moments. We had a disabled participant that used our facility often and he found it very difficult at our old location. I felt sad every time he came because it was so difficult for him to enter the building. It was a different story now. Not only did he have easier access, we also had a disabled access bathroom too. Yay!

There were also those days when it felt like we were walking through mud and making no progress, it was taking more time than I expected but the pieces were gradually coming together. It was a long third trimester. Ten months of fundraising and appealing to the community. Our community heard, people came forward and gave so much, in cash and in kind. I had not seen community generosity on this level before. When it was all said and done, we had reached in excess of $350,000 in cash and in kind.

Along the way a designer came on board offering her services pro bono. I loved the simple warm neutral colours and they worked really well in the space. We had asked for neutrals so that any seasonal decor would work, from Valentines to Christmas. Choosing a colour for the front door has fond memories too. I decided to go bright so I chose orange! It was shocking and beautiful and loud — it was hot! It was my way of giving a shout

out to all the kids who had sold cookies and buns to raise money for the door. Every time they passed the building the loud colour would "wave" to them.

The interior was gradually being completed. We loved the design. It gave the space a clean, sharp, fresh look. We replaced the blah, industrial-looking tin on the outside with a more attractive chocolate brown colour. It really stood out and made our logo look very cool. We moved the entrance of the building to the side where it made more sense for parents and kids, as the parking lot was on the side too.

After many months of renovations inside and out we were now ready for final inspections. It was time to get the overnight bag for the hospital ready; we had the list of all the things that would be needed after the birth. The suitcase needed to be packed and the trip to the hospital needed to be fully planned.

We started packing our things we were moving from the old building; it took a few days to pack and move all our possessions into a large trailer. It was a short distance but an epic move. We were finally saying goodbye to all that was familiar and leaving to embrace the future. Living this dream that no one thought would happen was about to begin. Thirty months of hoping, dreaming, imagining and envisioning what it would be like. Thirty months of carrying this baby was a long time, but we finally had a birth date in sight. It was fun and awkward, we were waddling a little and things were not perfect.

We discovered our limitations quickly as we unpacked. We did not have as much storage as we had hoped. The air conditioning needed programming, there were new lighting codes and missing keys, but we walked through it. It took almost a month to put things into the new space. As with all moves, this was a gradual process and it took time to bring everything in. We had packed up our old kitchen cabinets as they were still in good condition — we literally took them off the wall; the only thing we left was the kitchen sink in our old space. My staff team and I tackled the job of sanding and painting the old cupboards; it took us a few weeks to get that done. We bought new hardware and when it was all said and done we were able to meet some of our storage needs for reception, the training room, the playroom areas and one staff office, saving us in excess of $10,000.

Our original due date was August 12, 2014; we were more than two weeks overdue. Our water broke on September 7 and there was a buzz of activity as we started pushing. We finally "had our baby" on September 9, 2014. As expected we were nervous on day one; people were curious to see what the new building looked like and we needed to resume services for the families we served as soon as possible. We opened our doors to the general public and wouldn't you know it, some naysayers immediately pointed out our limitations. I chose to ignore the negative comments because they had not laboured, they had not carried this child, and they did not understand what it took. It was easy to complain and criticize a project, especially when you have not laboured or worked hard for it. This was like carrying a baby for nine months, bringing the baby home after thirty hours of labour pains and contractions and someone saying your child was ugly. It reminded me of the week I had Miqaela, I was proud as punch and at Sunday service when someone came up to me and asked if my daughter was homemade. Seriously? I just bit my tongue, hard.

I heard the comments and criticisms and took away only the constructive points. It was so funny that we had moved into this *safe* new facility with new bathrooms, a brand new kitchen with a ten-foot island, fully accessible — an absolutely phenomenal space — as well as three times the number of parking spaces we had previously, and the primary concern was there were no pictures on the wall! Go figure! I was so happy, it would not have mattered what anyone said. This baby was pretty!

There were growing pains, lots of them, and then there were the armchair quarterbacks who offered suggestions after the fact. They say the mountain does not grow bigger, you do. I grew in more ways than I could have imagined. We had a prime location, the best possible location for exposure; 15,000 cars passed our building daily. We were no longer hidden. As the saying goes, "Build it and they will come." I didn't know how they would come, but they came. Our participant numbers doubled in the first six months. The feedback was really good; moms told us they loved the new centre and it was obvious our kids enjoyed the new playroom. There was also a huge sense of accomplishment knowing that the community had come through for us. Together we had created a place where every family counts. Incidentally, the words "where every family counts" actually became our new tag line and is painted in huge letters on one of our largest walls.

The general public had now seen the building via the open house but Jocelyne was the first person I sent a personal invitation, as she had requested if we got the new building. It was an awesome day when she came. I took her on a tour of the building with so much pride. She was definitely impressed; I don't think she could believe how nice it was. She gave me a "this is insane, you actually it pulled it off" look. I understood, I had her respect and she had mine. What I was not expecting was what she did next. She pulled out her pocketbook and wrote us a cheque. She wished us all the very best. It meant a lot to me because Jocelyne really understood. We said our goodbyes and I went back to my office. It had been a long day; it was time to turn off the lights and go home. Just as I was about to leave my eye just caught the amount on Jocelyne's cheque — it was my turn to be shocked. There was only one thing I could say…this is CRAZY! Crazy has its rewards.

People

You can design and create, and build the most wonderful place in the world. But it takes people to make the dream a reality.

– Walt Disney

The one thing that links every chapter in this book is people. People are invaluable. Good people are priceless, period. There is no goal or dream that can be achieved without them. They are essential to any project or vision. They are an unparalleled resource in every life or business situation. I have been fascinated by people my whole life. I love the differences! From the diversity in our physical appearance to the diversity in the gifts we have all been endowed with, to our ability to make a difference when we work together to help one another. Nothing happens without people. My story, our centre's story, is rich with amazing people. Our story cannot be told without them, and nor can yours. I recall telling my boss that we did not need money to renovate, what we really needed were people. I was right.

I kept a picture of the families we served in my mind as I went out and talked about our cause to potential donors. I know many non-profit organizations/registered charities consider it difficult to raise funds, and the truth is it is difficult because no one wants to be turned down. Unfortunately it goes with the territory of running non-profit organizations. While fundraising for the new facility, I kept focused by connecting it to our purpose and people. It was an opportunity to tell our story over and over again. I really enjoyed doing that, I told our story with all the pride and joy I had and explained how much of a difference a few dollars could make. There were many times when I heard the word "no" more than I heard "yes" but I never stopped trying. I kept knocking on doors and when the going got tough and the freezing cold smacked my face and fingers I thought of Amber and I never gave up. You need to know your "why" and keep it front and centre. Ironically, what we were doing was helping people, and the only way to help those people was through help from other people. We were the bridge.

It would take a whole other book to tell you about our fundraising efforts and the support we got from the people in our community so I'll give you just a quick summary.

Our fundraising efforts began in late 2013. We put on concerts, bake sales, and perogy dinners, contests and silent auctions among many other events. I was particularly touched by little nine-year-old Susie who spent her summer operating a lemonade stand raising twenty dollars for us. I was so grateful for every dollar we received. Children, dads, moms, and grandparents alike were raising money for us in many different ways. Kids at a local school spent six months raising $400 by selling buns and cookies. I got the donation all in quarters! There were community barbecues, corporate dinners, a family even had a backyard drink-up and raised over $6000 for us. I should mention the day that I went into the radio station to give an interview appealing for donations. As I was driving away from the building after the segment, a truck followed me until he was able to flag down me down. He had heard the interview and wanted to give me a large cheque, which he did on the spot. I understood that our project needed people. Money is in human hands and the only way to get it, is to get people to give it.

We came to another tipping point early one morning in April. The building had already been gutted and framed by one of the contractors who had attended the breakfast meeting. We now had to look at the electrical plans. I did a walk through with an electrician; he said it would take two electricians two weeks to complete the work. Material and labour would be approximately $50,000. I was nervous as that would take up most of what we had left to buy all materials. I would be lying if I said I was not troubled. Donations were coming in but not at a fast rate. How was I going to foot the bill?

I got a call a few evenings later to meet the electricians at the new space early on a Tuesday morning. I wondered why, we had already gone over the figures and the plans. I arrived at 8:00 a.m. to a hub of activity, ten vans outside and there were eleven hefty guys running cables and wires throughout the new building. I was a little confused and concerned because I had not given a go-ahead for the work, we didn't have $50,000.

Brent, the owner of the electrical firm came up to me and explained that he was involved in fundraising the previous year for families in Mozambique and here I was trying to raise funds for moms and kids in his own backyard. He wanted to help. He said he offered his team a day off work or a day to volunteer wiring our building. His whole team showed up to volunteer! He was going to take care of all of our electrical needs for free! I don't cry easily but this brought tears to my eyes and relief to my heart! Good people huh? That one act of kindness brought so much validation and after much media coverage it started an avalanche of unprecedented donations to our organization. From that point on I could see that our project would be fully funded. We received paint, doors, kitchen cabinetry, appliances, lumber, decorative stone, trusses, lighting and much more.

There were so many instances when members of our community would come in and bring us all coffees or ice cream. Every gift was so very much appreciated because they kept us encouraged.

One afternoon after a particularly tiring and frustrating day I went to the bank before going to pick up the kids. An elderly gentleman came up to me; he must have been about eighty-five years old. He kept calling me Anna and even as I was explaining that my name was Vicki, he insisted. I thought it was a case of mistaken identity. He said his son was one of the workers at our site, and then the penny dropped. I said "Anna's House" and he beamed. Then he took a twenty-dollar bill out of his wallet and asked me to buy myself dinner. He wanted to pay for my meal. It touched my heart and encouraged me in a way that I cannot explain. It had the same impact as if he had given me $2000.

We were a testament to what people can do when they come together. I knew this was going to be a journey but this was crazy and a half! The power of people left me speechless.

I learned so many lessons about people. Treat everyone with respect regardless of who they are. Mary Kay Ash says, "Everyone has an invisible sign hanging from their neck saying, 'Make me feel important.' Never forget this message when working with people." I have always been a very grateful person; now I am even more so. Now that we had a "thank you" culture, our community also knew we were grateful. My staff team knows that even if someone gives us a paperclip, we express our appreciation immediately. I cannot say enough about the amazing staff team I have. A group of individuals that I can only describe as family, without them this could not have happened. They took care of our centre every day while I was out there pounding the pavements. They had the most amazing ideas and they believed (eventually) that we could accomplish our dream.

By September 2014, we were running a full-service family resource centre in a safe site. The renovations were almost completely paid for and the centre looked amazing. Most importantly families and especially children now had a safe place to grow because of the power of people.

Conclusion

Every story has an end but in life every end is just a new beginning.

– Anonymous

We finally had the baby and what a gorgeous baby it was. I dared to challenge life, I refused to back off, back down, turn off or turn down the sound of my dream and I won. "NO" just wasn't an option I was willing to accept.

My story wasn't without tears, frustration and raw pain. There is nothing pretty about my scars — mental, physical and emotional — but there is nothing that feels like winning. I understand the tears of elation that fall when you see the face on a newborn for the first time, when the child is placed on your chest and you hear that first cry. I experienced it personally and professionally. It's all the struggles, pain, pressure and near miscarriages along the way that make winning so special. I now have my two children and have helped bring an organization from a place of obscurity to a place of significance where it should be. What is really great for me is not just crossing the finishing line but winning and then going back to help others win too by writing this book. If anything, my journey so far has taught me to challenge the status the quo, never be reasonable, believe that the impossible is possible, stay crazy and if it is not broken, break it!

I am more excited now than when I began this book because I have grown so much in the process. It all starts with believing that you are crazy enough to have what you want. Go ahead and gather evidence and find stories of people who have done it and if you are the first then have the courage to be the first!

You have been on this journey with me, seen the highs and lows and some of the treacherous terrain I have had to cross. By now there should be no doubt that you can reach your dreams, and that craziness is an essential ingredient. The amount of craziness will depend on how wild your dreams are.

President Theodore Roosevelt said, "Far better is it to dare mighty things, to win glorious triumphs, even though checkered by failure... than to rank with those poor spirits who neither enjoy nor suffer much, because they live in a gray twilight that knows not victory nor defeat." This experience has awakened in me a quest to fight harder, dream bigger and climb higher on the crazy index! Thank you for the company along the way.

I will close Part Two as I began it in the words of Steve Jobs:

> "*Here's to the crazy ones. The misfits. The rebels. The troublemakers. The round pegs in the square holes. The ones who see things differently. They're not fond of rules. And they have no respect for the status quo. You can quote them,*

disagree with them, glorify or vilify them. About the only thing you can't do is ignore them. Because they change things. They push the human race forward. And while some may see them as the crazy ones, we see genius. Because the people who are crazy enough to think they can change the world, are the ones who do."

Now go out there, unleash your crazy and win!

A Message From the Author

Writing is like giving birth to a piano sideways. Anyone who perseveres is either talented or nuts.

– Flannery O'Connor

I have asked authors this question over and over, expecting a simple answer but never got it. Well it was now my turn to be asked I understand why. Recently someone asked "How on earth did you find the time to write a book with the schedule you have?" The simple answer is I didn't; I made the time. I typed it one letter at a time. Was it crazy? Yes. I agree with the quote by Flannery O'Connor above, nuts I am!

If something is important to you, you make time to do it. I have learned to hold time hostage by filling it with things that are meaningful to me as my comfort level with unfinished housework and homeless toys increases.

I also made a commitment to myself to write consistently and for me that was daily. There was sacrifice involved but the trade-off was worth it. I didn't have the luxury of a writing suite or a publisher's advance. I woke up early and many times that meant 3:45 a.m. (don't say crazy), and I went to work after that, but not before taking bread out of the oven, working out, waking kids up, making breakfast, packing lunches, getting the right sports kits, signing school journals, feeding the fish and dropping the kids off at daycare. There were days when I wrote pages and others when I barely wrote a paragraph; no matter what I just kept writing.

Martin Luther King Jr. said, "*If you can't fly, then run. If you can't run, then walk. If you can't walk, then crawl, but whatever you do you have to keep moving forward.*"

Trust me, I get the crawling, there were many days when all I did was crawl, but I kept moving.

I learned from the stories of so many others who dared to write their stories so I dared to write mine. I realize that we all have experiences and struggles and we can see pieces of our story in stories of others; I hope that sharing my story will help you see parts of your own story in mine and be encouraged to share your own.

I dreamed about writing it, wondered about it, imagined it, worried about it and I finally got to a place where I just had to sit my butt down and write it. I had wasted so much time and I couldn't sit for another minute longer, the book was bursting through everything I did. I couldn't silence the loud din of "doing nothing" so I did something about it. That loud voice in my head was quieted by the little clicking noise of my finger tapping away on my cell phone. No more Internet research or skimming through books or kits on how to write. The simple truth about how to write a book is to "just write," no drama, no thunder or lightning bolts, no deep soul searching or deep introspection. I simply picked up my phone and wrote my truth whenever and wherever I could.

As I am writing this piece I am actually waiting to see my chiropractor. Gone are the days when I moan at very long waiting times. I now use up all those minutes to write. My iPhone has a "notes" feature so every spare minute I can get I write. While standing in checkout lines, waiting in doctors' offices, waiting for rice to boil, sitting at long sporting events, and during plane stopovers I easily get pages done. My schedule is crazy for the most part and I continuously practice, or should I say juggle with the art and science of balance. Balance is tough, especially if you are a mom, wife, sister, auntie, team leader, chauffeur, sports mom, volunteer, domestic engineer and amateur nurse; like most moms, it takes practice. Being a single or solo parent makes it much harder but I actually became very resourceful when writing this book because I was able to "claim" all of my daily minutes that would otherwise have been wasted and turned them into this book. I wonder, how many books you have hidden in your day? I was really encouraged when I read about a very busy fifteen-hour-a-day UK lawyer and mother who turned her daily one-hour train commute into an e-book. You do what you have to do.

The only exception I have is basketball. I am a basketball nut. My son plays the game so no writing during his games. I am too busy screaming my head off supporting the team!

Ideas come in so many ways and I capture them as soon as possible. I either dictate them or type them into my phone. They say where there is a will there is a way, I found a way. My writing method is a little kamikaze and unorthodox but it works for me. This is my first iPhone-typed-book. I literally typed this whole book out on my iPhone 5 — all 50,000 words of it — and to think someone thought Steve Jobs was crazy... he was, I just built my crazy on top of his.

Having been on this journey with me you can see that being crazy is a great thing in fact and it is a necessary ingredient to do great things. According to Linda Rottenburg "Crazy is a compliment... if you have not been told your dream is crazy your dream is not big enough."

There is only one thing left to say; dream big and get lots of compliments!

Gratitude

This project would not have been completed without the help of so many people. It has taken a whole team of people to bring it from the basement to the bookshelf.

Thank you to God first of all for life itself and all it pertains. My faith has been an integral part of my journey and continues to be so.

Next is Victor, my knight in shining armour whose story I told quietly alongside mine, a rock, a friend, a lover and the best thing that ever happened to me on the earth. Without you I would not have had the courage and strength to fight all the battles we did. You are an awesome team mate! Sacrifice is a word that you lived out loud in front of me despite storms and tornados and tsunamis! You have soared high above the pressure and taught me how to soar too. Thank you for letting me tell so personal a story about you because you want to make a difference too. You said to me once many years ago. "To say I love you on day one is easy but saying it after many years there is a difference." This is twenty-one years later. I am still saying I love you! You are truly a strong but gentle giant. *Oluwa ni too to ti segun fun mi. A ba ara wa dale. Amin*

Miqaela & Michael, this is your story. You remind me every day when I see you that nothing is impossible and dreams are worth fighting for.

Liza "Jay" Adeyemi, Sis...thanks for being there always. PT, you never lived long enough to see all of your investment in me hit the bookstores. Thank you for challenging my thinking and for encouraging me to press on regardless. I am one of those in whom your legacy lives on. Pastor Tayo Adeyemi. Lived in Faith, died in faith 1962-2013.

Auntie Lola Odofin, what can I say? Your pikins love you plenty! MC Timmy & Lady G and baby Tim, we got next! The NASCAR team, thank you!

Mrs. V. A. Odofin, you are "never give up" personified. There are not enough pages to express my gratitude to you. I love you mum! Uncle and Auntie Bakare, *E seun.* My parents-in-law, the late Mr. & Mrs. Winston Olatundun, your love for me was special. I have treasured memories of you both. Thank you. *E sun re.*

Pastor Michael Olawore, thank you so much for your continued support. O3A, you know who you are, thank you for being my family no matter what. Yomi Ogunbiyi, *ore mi gidi*, thank you for hearing my endless chatting about the dream of writing this book and listening so intently as I read stuff over the phone. You have been there every step of the way. There is no friend like an old friend. Thank God for Excel!

Reena Nerbas, finally done! Your support has been priceless. You walked the path ahead of me and showed me where the potholes were. To my amazing staff team and the board of the Steinbach Family Resource Centre, thank you! My gratitude is immense, together we continue to make a difference. To the people of Steinbach, Manitoba thank you for being an example of what it means to be generous. Marcia Stewart, thank you for following your intuition. Judy Peters, thank you for fanning my crazy when there were only ashes of hope. Susan Fayinka, Mary Fayinka, Bim Alalade I know that you believed that I would get here, I finally have. The bracelet meant so much. Fumi P, It has been a long time coming but thankfully it is never too late to set a goal and achieve it. Done! Dr. Larry Dahl, I finally got it done, this dragon is slain, despite a few "sometimes's". You are a great mentor and dad. Thank you for being a voice of encouragement many times over. Kevin McFadden, your encouragement and support over the years have been priceless. Thank you for all you do to make the world a healthier place. Pastor Jeff and Susan Romas, Pastor Leon and Sally Fontaine, much love to you. Banjo Aromolaran-Eaton, thank you seems like such a small word. I owe you much. Love to little G.

Karl Phillips, you would not accept any excuse, nothing I could say would let me off the hook. Thank you for the constant support and encouragement and keeping me focused. 120, in all areas! You kept reminding me that I had what it took to succeed. Eric Thomas Ph.D., your story helped me tell mine. Beast mode! I can, I will, I have! CJ, this was the next level, I have mastered it, now I am moving on to the next one.

To my coach, Ryan Anderson, thank you for helping me challenge myself to reach my dreams. You are a great coach! You encourage, you support and you push. You are definitely one of the best! Persistence, Persistence, Persistence! Marnie Ferguson — Sarah was right, you are an amazing editor, you educated me in the process and you turned my words into a story worth reading. I literally threw a mud of writing at you and you turned it into reading pottery fit to be sold. I cannot thank you enough. Sarah Wood, you are a treasure to work with. Gary Blatz, everyone needs a graphic artist on their team, in you, I have the best!

Thank you to the many others who worked tirelessly behind the scenes and others who sent well wishes along the way. It has been a huge team effort and I am truly grateful.

Giving Back

I never got here by myself. So many people some of whom I will never meet have made sacrifices in various ways so that I could grow and learn and have choices I have. It is my honour to be able to give back to continue to improve the lives of others as others have done for me in my community. Thank you for joining me in this quest and making a contribution by buying this book. One dollar will be given to the Steinbach Family Resource Centre for every book sold to help cover program costs and look after families that use the centre. You are already a difference maker, please accept my sincere appreciation.

If you would like to make a donation to the centre please visit www.steinbachfrc.ca.

References:

Hallgren Roland, (1991). The Good Things in Life: A Study of the Traditional Religious Culture of the Yoruba People. *Lund Studies in African and Asian Religions 2*. Lund: Plus Ultra.

Koster-Oyekan ,Winny, (1999). Infertility among Yoruba Women: Perceptions on Causes, Treatments and Consequences, *African Journal of Reproductive Health*, *3*(1) pp. 13-26.

MacArthur, John, (1997). *MacArthur Study Bible,* Wheaton, IL: Good News Publishers, p. 25.

About the Author

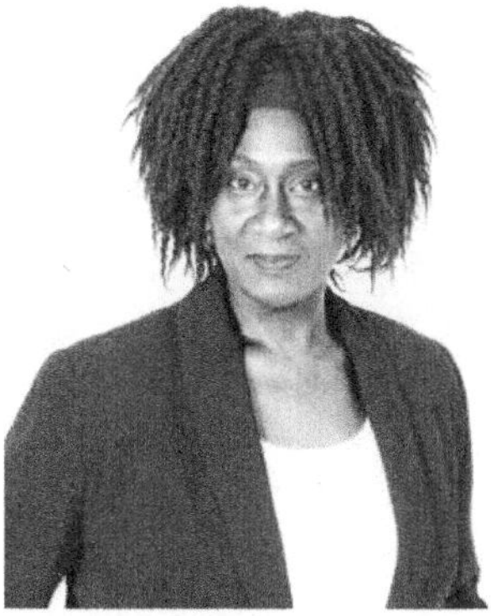

Vicki Olatundun is a persuasive, passionate, powerful high-octane motivational speaker. A socially conscious team leader with a passion for the people that she serves and the people she serves with. A former attorney turned social justice architect. She is known for her visionary abilities in the not-for-profit sector, the avenue through which she has been making a sustainable difference for those she serves over the last 15 years.

In 2014 Vicki was a nominee for the prestigious Woman of Distinction Award and in 2015 she was declared a "Change Maker," one of Canada's 40 women who are making Canada a better place by *Canadian Living Magazine.* A singer/songwriter, wife and mother to two adorable children, dubbed a DS by her seven-year-old son, a.k.a. Dragon Slayer. Vicki and her husband call Manitoba, their home where she is an executive director of a non-profit organization and is an instructor at a local college.

Vicki invites readers to e-mail her at VICKI@VICKIOLATUNDUN.COM.

Get lots more info at WWW.VICKIOLATUNDUN.COM.

Please look out for *Unleash Your Crazy To Win* audio and e-book coming soon.

Made in the USA
Coppell, TX
05 November 2026

11315624R00114